OXFORD HANDBOOKS
Series Editors R. N. Illingwo

D1434119

OXFORD HANDBOOKS IN EMERGENCY MEDICINE

This series has already established itself as the essential reference series for staff in A & E departments.

Each book begins with an introduction to the topic, including epidemiology where appropriate. The clinical presentation and the immediate practical management of common conditions are described in detail, enabling the casualty officer or nurse to deal with the problem on the spot. Where appropriate a specific course of action is recommended for each situation and alternatives discussed. Information is clearly laid out and easy to find—important for situations where swift action may be vital.

Details on when, how, and to whom to refer patients are covered, as well as the information required at referral, and what this information is used for. The management of the patient after referral to a specialist is also outlined.

The text of each book is supplemented with checklists, key points, clear diagrams illustrating practical procedures, and recommendations for further reading.

The Oxford Handbooks in Emergency Medicine are an invaluable resource for every member of the A & E team, written and edited by clinicians at the sharp end.

Emergency Management of Hand Injuries

G. R. Wilson
Consultant Hand Surgeon,
Queen Mary's University Hospital, Roehampton, London

P. A. Nee
Consultant in Accident and Emergency Medicine
Whiston Hospital, Merseyside

J. S. Watson
Consultant Hand Surgeon,
Withington Hospital, Manchester

Illustrated by R. K. Harrison
Chief Medical Artist,
Withington Hospital, Manchester

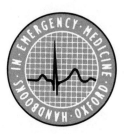
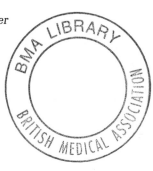

Oxford • New York • Tokyo
OXFORD UNIVERSITY PRESS
1997

Oxford University Press, Great Clarendon Street, Oxford OX2 6DP,
Oxford   New York
Athens   Auckland   Bangkok   Bogota   Bombay   Buenos Aires
Calcutta   Cape Town   Dar es Salaam   Delhi   Florence   Hong Kong
Istanbul   Karachi   Kuala Lumpur   Madras   Madrid   Melbourne
Mexico City   Nairobi   Paris   Singapore   Taipei   Tokyo   Toronto
and associated companies in
Berlin   Ibadan

Oxford is a trade mark of Oxford University Press

Published in the United States
by Oxford University Press Inc., New York

A catalogue record for this book is available from the British Library

Library of Congress Cataloging in Publication Data

Wilson, G. R. (Geoffrey Ross)
Emergency management of hand injuries / G. R. Wilson, P. A. Nee,
J. S. Watson; illustrated by R. K. Harrison.
(Oxford handbooks in emergency medicine; 17)
Includes bibliographical references and index.
1. Hand—Wounds and injuries—Handbooks, manuals, etc.
I. Nee, P. A.   II. Watson, J. S. (James Stewart)   III. Title.   IV. Series.
[DNLM: 1. Hand Injuries—therapy—handbooks.   2. Hand Injuries—
diagnosis—handbooks.   3. Emergencies—handbooks.   WB 39 098 v. 17
1997]
RD559.W55   1997
617.5'75044—dc20
DNLM/DLC   for Library of Congress   96–35095   CIP

ISBN 0 19 262824 0 (Hbk)
ISBN 0 19 262823 2 (Pbk)

Typeset by Footnote Graphics, Warminster, Wilts
Printed in Great Britain by
Bookcraft Ltd., Midsomer Norton, Avon

Contents

vi • Contents

Part 1

General considerations

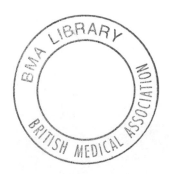

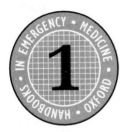

CHAPTER 1

Introduction

Patients with hand injuries or non-traumatic disorders of the hand commonly present to accident and emergency (A&E) departments. Although rarely life threatening in themselves, such injuries are the cause of considerable morbidity and loss of earnings. The majority are assessed initially by junior doctors in the A&E department where injuries may be overlooked or their severity underestimated.

Many hand conditions can be satisfactorily managed by junior A&E doctors, whilst others require input from more senior practitioners. At the more severe end of the spectrum are injuries that should be referred to a hand surgeon, either orthopaedic or plastic. A surgeon dedicated to the speciality will achieve better results than the occasional surgeon. The problems associated with operative procedures in the A&E department are many: a busy harassed casualty officer, a small operating area with poor lighting, inadequate instrumentation, and variable support from hand therapists.

The management of hand injuries has changed in recent years with more emphasis on anatomical reduction of fractures, where appropriate, and intensive follow up by trained Hand Therapists. No 'standard' treatment exists for a given injury, the management plan is determined by a number of factors including the age, handedness and occupation of the injured person as well as hobbies, pastimes, patient-preference and motivation.

The hand specialist aims to minimise symptoms and optimise function after an injury. The quality of treatment provided in an A&E department impacts significantly on outcome for many hand-injured patients.

This book has been written by two hand surgeons and an A&E specialist. It is not intended to be a comprehensive textbook but rather a pocket-sized manual which is easy to carry and easy to access. We aim to bridge the gap between the brief departmental guidelines, usually provided by the orthopaedic service, and the larger textbooks. The book covers the initial assessment and treatment of common injuries and disorders of the hand. It will benefit junior doctors with little experience in hand surgery who are nevertheless expected to manage such conditions on a daily basis.

Further reading
Lister, G. *The hand diagnosis and indications.* (1993). 3rd edition. Churchill Livingstone.

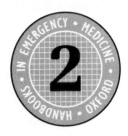

CHAPTER 2

Abbreviations

AbPB	abductor pollicis brevis
AbPL	abductor pollicis longus
AP	antero-posterior
ASB	anatomical snuff box
CMCJ	carpo-metacarpal joint
DIPJ	distal interphalangeal joint
DP	distal phalanx
ECRB	extensor carpi radialis brevis
ECRL	extensor carpi radialis longus
EDC	extensor digitorum communis
EDM	extensor digiti minimi
EIP	extensor indicis proprius
EPB	extensor pollicis brevis
EPL	extensor pollicis longus
FB	foreign body
FDP	flexor digitorum profundus
FDS	flexor digitorum superficialis
FPL	flexor pollicis longus
GA	general anaesthetic
IPJ	interphalangeal joint
IVFR	intravenous fluid resuscitation
LA	local anaesthetic
MC	metacarpal
MPJ	metacarpophalangeal joint
MP	middle phalanx
NAI	non-accidental injury
ORIF	open reduction and internal fixation
PIPJ	proximal interphalangeal joint
PMH	past medical history

PL	palmaris longus
POP	plaster of Paris
PP	proximal phalanx
PRBC	packed red blood cells
UCL	ulnar collateral ligament
#	fracture

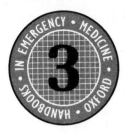

CHAPTER 3

Anatomy

Key points in anatomy

- Bones and joints
- Muscles and tendons
- Arteries and veins
- Nerves
- Skin, nails, and spaces

Knowledge of some basic anatomy of the hand is essential. It will help in the diagnosis of injuries and also in communication when referring the patient.

By convention the upper limb is divided into arm from shoulder to elbow, forearm from elbow to wrist, wrist, and hand. The anterior surface is usually termed **volar** and the posterior surface **dorsal** (Fig. 3.1). Rather than lateral and medial, which may cause some confusion, it is better to refer to radial (towards the thumb) and ulnar (towards the little finger). The digits should be called by their names and not by numbers, i.e. **thumb, index, middle** (or long), **ring**, and **little**. For descriptive purposes the fingers can be divided into proximal, middle, and distal compartments (proximal and distal in the thumb). Some hand surgeons use the mid-lateral line as a surgical approach. This is drawn with the finger flexed (Fig. 3.2).

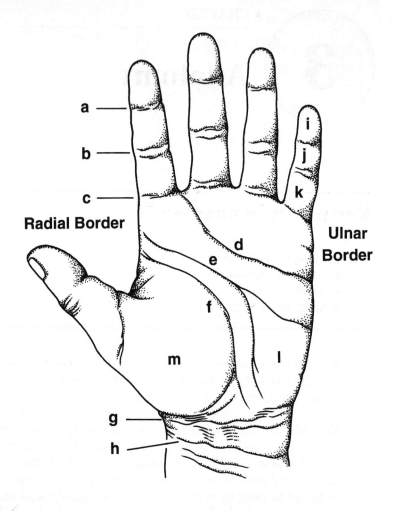

Radial Border

Ulnar Border

a DIPJ crease
b PIPJ crease
c palmar digital crease
d distal palmar crease
e proximal palmar crease
f thenar crease
g distal wrist crease
h proximal wrist crease
i distal segment (or compartment)
j middle segment
k proximal segment
l hypothenar eminence
m thenar eminence

Fig. 3.1 • Volar surface of the left hand.

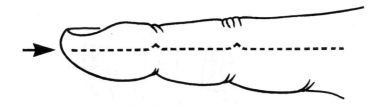

Fig. 3.2 ● Mid-lateral line of the finger, (arrow). ⋆

Bones and joints

The bones and joints are described in Figs. 3.3. The volar plate is a thickening of the joint capsule. It is one of the structures that limit hyperextension of the joint.

Muscles and tendons

Flexors

There are two long flexor tendons to each finger: the flexor digitorum superficialis (FDS) which is attached to the base of the middle phalanx and flexes the PIPJ, and the flexor digitorum profundus (FDP) which is attached to the base of the distal phalanx and flexes the DIPJ. The hand is divided descriptively into five zones based on the relationship of the tendons to each other and to other structures (Fig. 3.4). Lacerations distal to the PIPJ crease of the finger will probably divide only the FDP tendon, whereas a laceration more proximally may divide one or both tendons. The flexor tendons run within a sheath in the digits. This sheath has thickenings which act as pulleys; the most important are the A2 and A4 pulleys

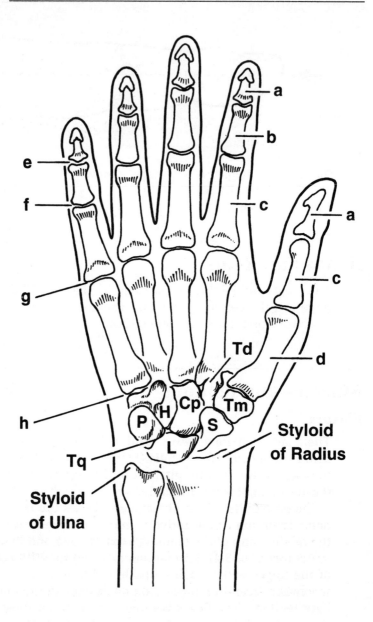

Fig. 3.3 • (a) Bones and joints of the hand and wrist;

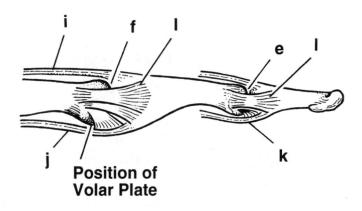

**Position of
Volar Plate**

a	terminal (distal) phalanx	k	FDP
b	middle phalanx	l	collateral ligament
c	proximal phalanx	Tm	trapezium
d	metacarpal	Td	trapezoid
e	DIPJ	Cp	capitate
f	PIPJ	H	hamate
g	MCPJ	P	pisiform
h	CMCJ	Tq	triquetral
i	central slip of EDC	L	lunate
j	FDS	S	scaphoid

Fig. 3.3 • (*cont.*) (b) lateral view of digit.

(Fig. 3.5). The thumb has one long flexor, flexor pollicis longus (FPL), which is attached to the base of the distal phalanx and flexes the IPJ.

There are three thenar muscles at the base of the thumb which can oppose and abduct the thumb and flex the MPJ. These are supplied by the median nerve (there are three similar muscles to the little finger supplied by the ulnar nerve). In the palm is the adductor pollicis, also supplied by the ulnar nerve, which approximates the thumb towards the palm.

Between the metacarpal bones are the interosseous muscles. The three palmar interossei adduct the fingers

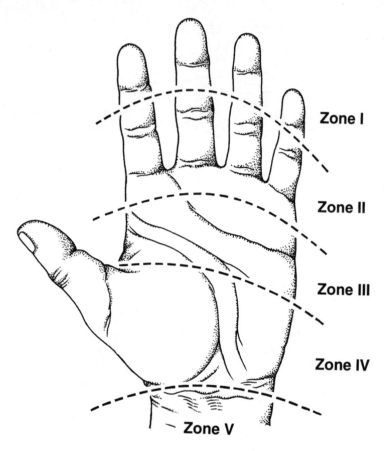

Fig. 3.4 • Zones of flexor tendon injuries in the hand and wrist.

(relative to the middle finger, so that there are none to the middle finger) and the four dorsal interossei abduct the fingers away from the axis of the middle finger (so that the middle finger has two). The little finger has its own abductor. It is easy to test the bulk and action of the first dorsal interosseous, the last muscle supplied by the ulnar nerve (Fig. 3.6).

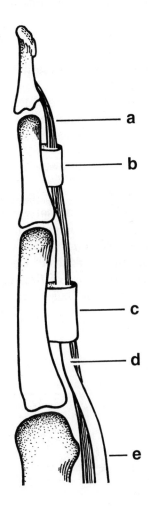

a FDP tendon
b A4 pulley attached to middle phalanx
c A2 pulley attached to proximal phalanx
d decussation of FDS
e FDS tendon

Fig. 3.5 • A2 and A4 pulleys: thickenings of the flexor sheath.

The four lumbricals are unusual muscles in that they take origin from and are inserted into tendons. They run from the FDP tendons in the palm to the extensor tendons on the back of the fingers. They act like tensioners and allow the fingers to remain straight whilst the MPJs are flexed (Fig. 3.7).

The other tendons on the volar aspect of the wrist are flexor carpi ulnaris (FCU), palmaris longus (sometimes absent), and flexor carpi radialis (FCR) (Fig. 3.8).

Extensors

The extensor tendons to the thumb form the anatomical snuff box. The EPL lies dorsally and inserts into the base of the distal phalanx—it extends the IPJ of the thumb. The AbPL and EPB tendons lie volarly and abduct and extend the thumb metacarpal. Deep in the snuff box are the two radial extensors of the wrist (ECRL and ECRB) which insert into the bases of the second and third metacarpals. The ECU tendon is the most ulnar of the

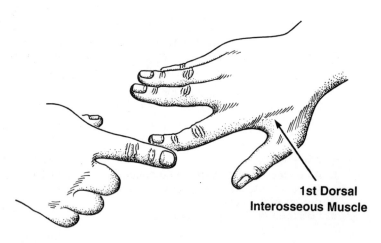

**1st Dorsal
Interosseous Muscle**

Fig. 3.6 • Tensing first dorsal interosseous muscle (ulnar nerve).

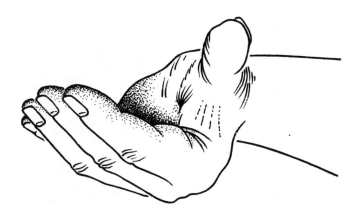

Fig. 3.7 ● Action of lumbrical muscles.

extensor tendons and inserts into the base of the fifth metacarpal (Fig. 3.9). The action of the extensors to the fingers is quite complex. There are two extensors to the index (EDC and EIP) and little fingers (EDC and EDM), and only one each to the middle and ring fingers (EDC). The extensor tendons fan out across the back of the hand. Their main action is to extend the MCP joints. As the tendons pass over the MCP joints they are stabilized by tough transverse fibres known as the sagittal bands. Over the proximal compartments of the fingers the tendon divides into a central slip and two lateral slips. The latter are joined by slips from the lumbricals and interossei. The central slip inserts into the base of the middle phalanx and extends the PIPJ, while the two lateral slips pass around the PIPJ to insert into the base of the distal phalanx and extend both the PIPJ and the DIPJ.

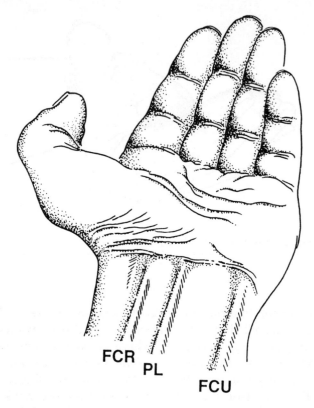

Fig. 3.8 • Volar aspect of wrist.

Arteries and veins

The arterial supply to the hand is derived largely from the radial and ulnar arteries. At the wrist the radial artery lies on the radial side of the FCR tendon. Its main branch then passes beneath the thumb extensors within the anatomical snuff box. It pierces the muscles between the thumb and index finger to come to lie on the volar aspect of the palm and then forms the palmar arch by uniting with the terminal branch of the ulnar artery.

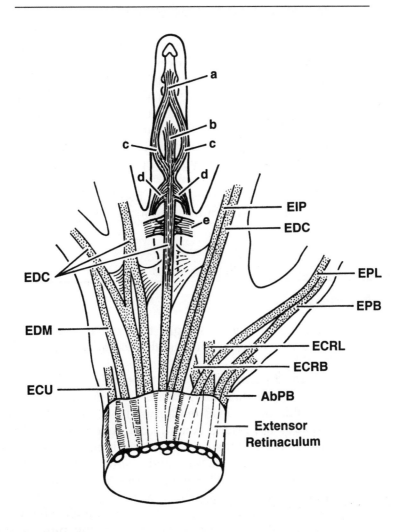

a extensor insertion into distal phalanx
b central slip
c lateral slip
d slips from lumbrical and interossei
e saggital bands

Fig. 3.9 • Position of the extensor tendons on the dorsum of the hand and fingers.

The ulnar artery lies just radial to the FCU tendon running with the ulnar nerve; it passes radial to the pisiform bone and its main branch turns across the palm to join the arch from the radial artery.

The fingers have two digital arteries derived from the palmar arch. Each passes along the lateral borders of the fingers just dorsal and deep to the digital nerves. The blood supply to the thumb is complex. It arises mainly from branches off the radial artery. There are two main arteries on the volar aspect of each side of the thumb.

The majority of veins in the hand are on the dorsum. They drain mostly into the cephalic and basilic veins in the forearm.

Nerves

The classical nerve supply to the hand is described (Fig. 3.10). There is considerable variation between individuals.

There are two major and three minor nerves to the hand. The **median** nerve passes through the wrist on the ulnar side of the FCR tendon under cover of PL tendon when this is present. About 3 cm proximal to the distal wrist crease it sends a small palmar branch which passes above the carpal tunnel and supplies skin over the thenar eminence. The main nerve passes through the carpal tunnel beneath the flexor retinaculum and into the palm. It then sends off a motor branch which supplies the thenar muscles before dividing into sensory branches to the thumb, index, and middle fingers and half the ring finger. Through these sensory branches it also supplies the first (or first and second) lumbrical.

The **ulnar** nerve runs in the wrist just radial to the FCU tendon, between the tendon and the ulnar artery. It passes into a canal on the radial side of the pisiform bone and then divides in the palm. The sensory branch

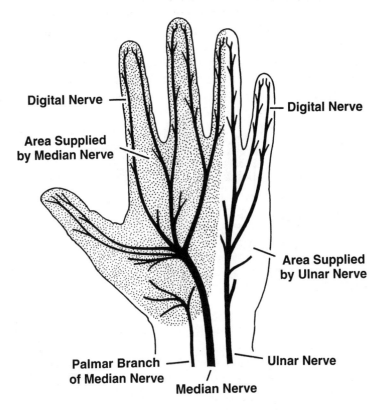

Fig. 3.10 • Nerve supply to the volar aspect of the hand.

supplies the little finger and half the ring finger. The motor branch supplies all the interossei, and the ulnar supplies two or three lumbricals, the hypothenar muscles, and the adductor pollicis. A dorsal branch of the ulnar nerve arises 3–4 cm proximal to the distal wrist crease. It supplies the ulnar side of the dorsum of the hand and the dorsum of the little finger and half the ring finger.

The **radial** nerve at the wrist is purely sensory. It runs radial to the radial artery and then over the tendons of the snuff box. It supplies an area on the dorsal surfaces of the hand, thumb, index, and middle fingers and half the ring finger as far distally as the middle compartments (Fig. 3.11).

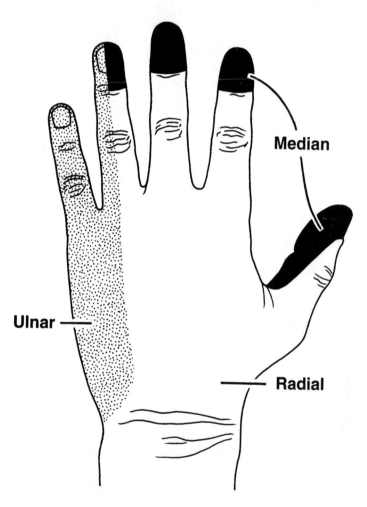

Fig. 3.11 ● Sensory nerve distribution on the dorsal surface of left hand.

Each finger has two main **digital** nerves which run on the volar aspect of each digit laterally. Each supplies half of the digit on the volar aspect and also the dorsal surface of the distal compartment.

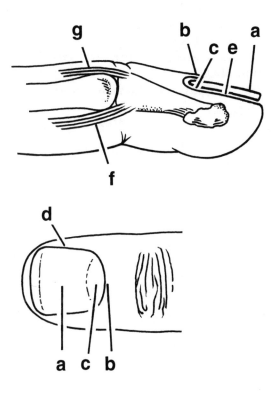

a nail plate
b eponychium (nail fold)
c lunula (overlies germinal matrix)
d paronychium
e sterile matrix (nail bed)
f insertion of FDP
g insertion of extensor tendon

Fig. 3.12 ● Fingertip and nail.

Skin, nails, spaces

The volar skin is bound down and relatively fixed. The dorsal skin is more elastic and mobile. The volar surface has a number of creases that are approximately related to underlying joints (Fig. 3.1).

The main features of the nail are shown in Fig. 3.12.

There are a number of spaces in the hand that are important because they can become infected. The main areas where abscesses can form are finger pulp, flexor tendon sheaths, the thenar and hypothenar spaces, the mid-palm space, and the web spaces.

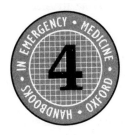

CHAPTER 4

Assessment

Key points in assessment
- History – Listen to the patient
- General examination
- Specific examination

Key points in specific examination
- Look
- Feel
- Move
- X-ray

When a patient presents with an injury to the hand it is essential to take an adequate history and carry out a thorough examination if injuries and complications are not to be overlooked. It is possible to carry out a fairly comprehensive examination of the hand in a very short time if a well-practised systematic approach is employed. The principles of **look, feel, move, X-ray** apply. When the hand is injured, have a low threshold for ordering an X-ray.

It is useful to assess overall function first ('make a fist', 'straighten your fingers') and then go on to consider potential complications of the presenting injury and specifically test for them. For example: 'What structures lie beneath this laceration?'

The patient may have to be encouraged to demonstrate his full range of movement because of pain. Systemic analgesia is appropriate for more severe injuries, but avoid local anaesthesia until the patient has been assessed by someone senior.

When testing for evidence of bony injury it is possible to stress the injured part by applying pressure remote from associated soft tissue swelling which will inevitably be tender.

Remember to examine the joints proximal and distal to any injured joint.

Record all positive and important negative signs (e.g. 'sensation normal') using appropriate nomenclature.

History

'Listen to the patient': he often knows what is wrong with his hand—whether it feels numb, or whether he can move it.

The history should include the following points under three main headings.

The patient

- Age, sex, handedness, occupation.
- Relevant pastimes/hobbies, e.g. musician.
- Previous illnesses/injuries/operations on the relevant limb.
- Current medications, allergies, tetanus status, time of last meal.

Mechanism of injury

- Attitude of hand when injured.
- Protective devices (e.g. machine guard, gloves).
- Nature of injuring forces:
  Name of machine.
  What (exactly) does it do?

Which part (describe) caused the injury?
Was there entrapment, and for how long?
What was the normal size of the gap within which
the hand was trapped?
Was there heat involved?
How was the hand released?

- Blood loss at scene: enquire of ambulance personnel or
other witness.

Present symptoms

- Pain, numbness, weakness.

Listen to the patient

Examination

There are three important aspects of your examination:

General examination

- Distress, colour (pallor, cyanosis), signs of hypo-
volaemia?
- Baseline observations—pulse, blood pressure, respira-
tory rate.
- In the context of major trauma the initial assessment
and resuscitation of the patient should be conducted
in accordance with ATLS guidelines.
- Are there any associated injuries?
- Carry out a complete secondary survey and appropriate radiology.

Injured hand—general

- **Look:** Examine the front and back of the hand for
colour, swelling deformity, wounds, and normal cascade of fingers (Fig. 4.1).
- **Feel** Bony tenderness, crepitus, instability.
- **Move:** Active and passive range of movement, e.g.
full curl-up (the ability to approximate the fingernails
to the palm).

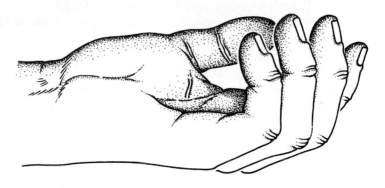

Fig. 4.1 • Normal 'cascade' of fingers in the relaxed position.

Injured hand—specific

Tendons
Evaluate specific tendons as below. Beware the partially divided tendon – pain on movement is not a reliable sign.

FDS
Ask the patient to bend the finger while you hold the other fingers in full extension (thereby inactivating the deep flexors). The DIPJ should be flaccid; this is particularly important when testing the FDS of the index finger as the FDP to index may be independent of the other deep flexors (Fig. 4.2).

FDP
Ask the patient to bend the tip of the finger (DIPJ) while you hold the PIPJ straight (Fig. 4.3).

Extensor tendons
Ask the patient to straighten the fingers. This will test the long extensors which straighten the MPJs. Extension at the PIPJ can be effected by intrinsic muscles of the hand (lumbricals and interossei). Straightening the

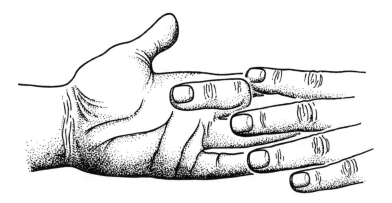

Fig. 4.2 • Testing FDS.

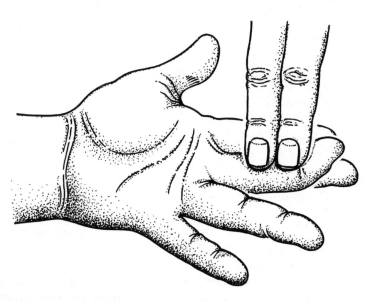

Fig. 4.3 • Testing FDP.

fingers against resistance, with your index finger pushing on the dorsum of the proximal phalanx, will test the strength of the extensors.

FPL
Hold the proximal compartment of the thumb between your thumb and index finger and ask the patient to bend the thumb (at the IPJ).

EPL
Ask the patient to touch your finger with his thumb. With the hand palm down on a flat surface, the EPL tendon will stand out when the thumb is elevated. Palpate the tendon of EPL.

Nerves
Test for specific nerve injury as below. Beware partial division and delayed loss of function. If a nerve injury is a possibility, review the patient in a day or two.

Digital nerves
There is a digital nerve running down each side of the digit. The best objective test for nerve integrity is the presence of sweating. When a nerve is cut, sweating stops in about 4 minutes, and sweat is needed for normal grip. When a plastic ball-point pen is rubbed down the side of a finger there should be some resistance. When there is no sweating (nerve injury), the finger is smooth and the pen glides very easily. This is a surprisingly reliable test.

You can test for light touch, but this is very subjective—especially in an injured hand!

Median nerve
The median nerve has motor and sensory functions.

Sensory—the nerve supplies the thumb and the radial two and a half digits. Its palmar branch supplies sensation to the radial half of the palm. Test for sweating in the relevant digits.

Motor—the nerve supplies the thenar muscles (not adductor pollicis) and the first lumbrical. Test AbPB by asking the patient to elevate the thumb against resis-

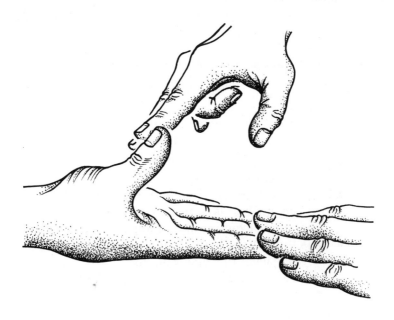

Fig. 4.4 • Testing AbPB (median nerve).

tance, with the palm-up hand flat on the table. Palpate the muscles of the thenar eminence (Fig. 4.4).

Ulnar nerve
The ulnar nerve also has motor and sensory functions.

Sensory—the nerve supplies the ulnar one and a half digits. There is a dorsal branch that supplies the ulnar side of the back of the hand and the ulnar one and a half digits.

Motor—the nerve supplies all the other muscles in the hand. Test by resisted abduction of the index while feeling the bulk of the first dorsal interosseous muscle with the index finger of your other hand (Fig. 3.6). Alternatively ask the patient to place the hand palm down on a flat surface, hyperextend the middle finger only, and then wiggle the finger from side to side.

Radial nerve

This is purely a sensory nerve in the hand. It supplies an area on the dorsum of the hand, radially and onto the backs of the thumb and the radial two and a half digits. Testing the sweat is not very useful here (as there are not many sweat glands). Test for light touch or pinprick.

Circulation

Do the hand and fingers have a *proper* blood supply? It can be difficult to assess the circulation to the hand, and this examination must not be cursory.

- Note the colour (of 'normal' side). Pale? Blue?
- Palpate the ulnar and radial pulses.
- Are the fingers as warm as the fingers on the other hand, or adjacent uninjured fingers?
- Does the patient have normal sensation? Most arteries travel adjacent to a major nerve.
- Is there a normal capillary return? Press the fingertip or nail and watch for the speed of return of the blush— it should take less than 2 seconds in a warm room (as long as it takes you to say 'capillary return time').

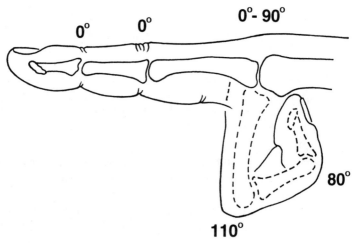

Fig. 4.5 • Normal range of joint movements.

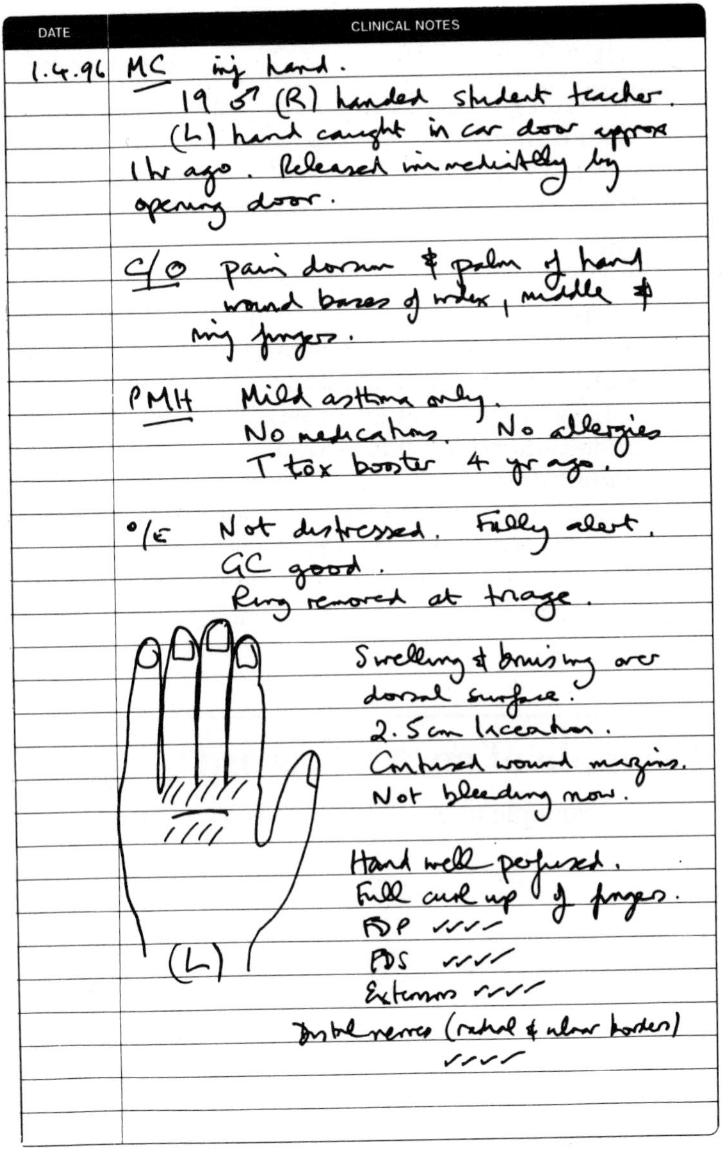

DATE	CLINICAL NOTES

1.4.96 MC inj hand.

19 y° (R) handed student teacher.
(L) hand caught in car door approx
1 hr ago. Released immediately by
opening door.

C/O pain dorsum & palm of hand
wound bases of index, middle &
ring fingers.

PMH Mild asthma only.
No medications. No allergies
T tox booster 4 yr ago.

O/E Not distressed. Fully alert.
GC good.
Ring removed at triage.

Swelling & bruising over
dorsal surface.
2.5 cm laceration.
Contused wound margins.
Not bleeding now.

Hand well perfused.
Full curl up of fingers.
FDP ✓✓✓
FDS ✓✓✓
Extensors ✓✓✓
Dbl nerves (radial & ulnar borders)
✓✓✓

(L)

Fig. 4.6 ● A&E record.

- The most reliable test is the turgor in the fingertip. Squeeze the fingertip; the pulp should refill immediately. If it stays squashed, there is no effective circulation.

The finger may have an adequate arterial input but no venous drainage. The finger will be warm, possibly with normal sensation, but it will be swollen with a bluish coloration. The capillary return will be very rapid.

Joints

Test the range of movements of the joints. If the range is normal you can record 'full extension and curl-up'. If there is reduced movement (compared with the uninjured hand), record the range of movement (Fig. 4.5). If there is a greater range of passive movement than active movement record this as well.

Stability: stress the joint between your finger and thumb trying to move the distal component off the axis of the digit (in lateral and AP planes). There should be very little if any movement. If there is excessive 'travel', compare with the normal side as some people's joints can be very lax.

Example of an A&E record

An example of an A&E record is shown in Fig. 4.6.

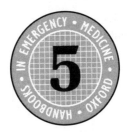

CHAPTER 5

Surgery, splints, and dressings

Key points in surgery, splints, and dressings

- Tourniquet for most surgical procedures
- Elevate in a sling
- Tetanus status

Surgery in the A&E department

Many limitations to practising surgery on the hand are imposed by the average A&E department—lack of space, poor choice of instrumentation and magnification, pressure of work, poor lighting, no hand table, and problems of follow-up and rehabilitation. This is why it is suggested throughout the text that many procedures are carried out by the hand service rather than in the A&E department. Most procedures carried out in A&E can be performed adequately under local anaesthetic. However, not all patients can cope with this, and so very occasionally a patient may require a general anaesthetic.

Tourniquet

A bloodless field is essential for all but the simplest laceration. Most patients can tolerate a pneumatic tourniquet for a short period, especially on the forearm. Proprietary exsanguinating digital tourniquets (e.g. Tourni-cot, Mar Med, Michigan) are ideal for single-

For procedures carried out in the A&E department the following instruments should be available as a minimum on a 'hand set'.

1. Stable Hand Table
2. Loupe magnification
3. Scalpel with a no. 15 blade
4. Two skin hooks
5. Two catspaw retractors
6. Fine dissecting forceps (Adson's)
7. Scissors:
   curved enucleation scissors
   dressing scissors
8. Syringe (to irrigate the wound)
9. Fine-needle holder (Halsey)
10. Bipolar diathermy (or fine absorbable ties)
11. Skin suture, 4/0 or 5/0 monofilament (e.g. Ethilon, Novafil)

finger injuries. Alternatively, an examining finger stall or the finger of a surgical glove with the tip cut off can be rolled down the (anaesthetized) finger to act as exsanguinator and tourniquet. Never use a narrow rubber tube and clip as the pressure beneath this can be very high.

Dressings

Does the patient need a dressing? Many wounds are best left exposed. As long as a synthetic monofilament suture has been used, the patient can later gently wash the wound with soap and water and dab it dry with a towel.

Some patients are uncomfortable without a dressing. A sticking plaster may be all that is needed. This is unlikely to interfere with mobility.

For larger dressings, a layer or two of tulle gras will reduce the adhesion of the dressing when it needs to be changed. There is no evidence that the antibiotic- or antiseptic-impregnated tulles have any advantage over plain tulle gras.

Cotton gauze will absorb any exudate and will distribute the pressure of the bandage evenly. If the gauze is moistened with sterile saline, this will improve absorption and prevent adhesion. A crepe bandage holds the dressing in place. The patient must be warned of the signs and symptoms of a tight dressing, i.e. increasing pain, numbness, colour change of the fingers (blue or white). Written advice may be useful.

Tubegauz on a metal applicator is useful for individual finger dressings. Be careful not to overtwist it as it is applies, as this can cause a tourniquet effect.

Small burns are dressed with tulle gras and gauze or a semipermeable membrane dressing (e.g. Opsite, Tegaderm). Larger areas should be referred to the hand surgeon or burns unit. They are often dressed in a Flamazine bag. The hand is smeared with Flamazine (silver sulphadiazine), and placed in a polythene bag. This is bandaged at the wrist, with some gauze placed between the bag and the skin of the wrist to absorb the exudate. Encourage the patient to mobilize his fingers in the bag.

After the dressing is applied, ELEVATE IN A SLING.

Immobilization

Does the hand need to be immobilized? Many injuries including stable fractures are best elevated and mobilized. This reduces swelling and stiffness.

A simple bandage on the hand does nothing for the injury, but will remind the patient and others that the hand is injured. Many patients feel happier with a bandage on an injured hand.

Most significant injuries will benefit from a period of elevation and immobilization. A plaster of Paris slab is a good way of immobilizing an injured hand. The slab is usually applied to the volar surface, with the hand in the safe position (Fig. 5.1). The wrist is comfortably extended, with the MPJs at 70°–90°, and the IPJs at 0°–15°.

The **mallet splint** was designed to treat mallet injuries of the fingers. It may be useful to treat other injuries of the finger tip. It is imperative that the PIPJ is allowed free movement, and is not taped down (Fig. 5.2).

A **foam-backed aluminium splint** (e.g. Zimmer) is useful for immobilizing parts of the hand, while allowing the rest of the hand to mobilize. It is applied with the foam side against the skin and is bent into the desired shape. The ends should be bent back and the corners trimmed, as they can be very sharp. It is also important to avoid the tourniquet effect of circumferential strapping. MP joints should be held at 70°–90°, and IP joints at 0°–15°. When immobilizing a joint, the adjacent joints should be free to mobilize if the injury allows this.

Buddy Strapping (neighbour strapping) is useful for painful fingers and stable fractures. It keeps the IPJs mobile and encourages movement in the injured digit whilst preventing lateral stress (Fig. 5.3). The injured digit is strapped to an adjacent finger of similar size, with a small piece of cotton gauze between the digits.

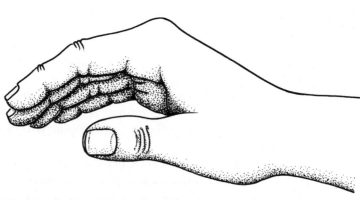

Fig. 5.1 • Safe position for hand immobilisation.

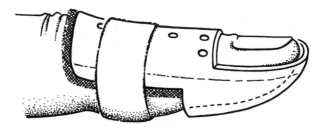

Fig. 5.2 ● Stack mallet splint.

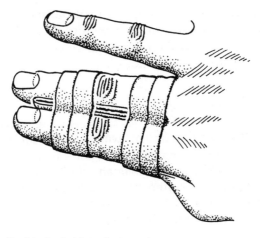

Fig. 5.3 ● Buddy (neighbour) strapping.

Antitetanus

Your department will have an antitetanus policy. With a significant or severely contaminated wound in a non immune patient give 500 units of human antitetanus immunoglobulin in addition to antitetanus toxoid (inject at a different site), plus a 5-day course of oral penicillin V.

Antibiotics

There is no indication for routine antibiotic prophylaxis. The indications for use of antibiotics are:

- an open joint
- an open fracture
- a bite wound
- a contaminated wound
- an 'old' wound (more than 12 hours before it receives any treatment)
- a patient with no tetanus immunity

Abscesses need incision and drainage, although a surrounding cellulitis may need antibiotics.

The best treatment for a wound is debridement of any dead tissue and then thorough lavage of the wound with at least 500 ml of saline.

Examples of appropriate antibiotics.
- **Cellulitis:** IV benzyl penicillin for 24–48 hours then oral penicillin with or without flucloxacillin (erythromycin if allergic to penicillin)
- **Staphylococcal infection** (boil, paronychia): flucloxacillin (erythromycin if allergic to penicillin)
- **Bite:** amoxycillin plus metronidazole or co-amoxiclav
- **Open fracture or joint:** flucloxacillin in or cefuroxime

---

Ring Removal

All rings should be removed from an injured hand. Some swelling is inevitable. Warm soapy water may suffice. Other techniques using tape or twine have been described. We have found it preferable to 'milk' the swollen tissues under the ring in a proximal direction. Sometimes it is necessary to use a ring cutter.

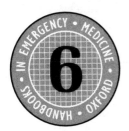

CHAPTER 6

Local anaesthetic techniques

Key points in local anaesthetic techniques

- A second doctor must be available when you perform Bier's block
- Do not use Bier's block unless you are competent in managing any complications
- Avoid lignocaine with adrenaline for digital nerve blocks
- Use a 27G needle for nerve blocks
- Do not try to elicit paraesthesiae, intraneural canulation causes neuroma.

Many minor hand surgical procedures can be carried out under local anaesthetic in the A&E department.

Lignocaine is the usual anaesthetic used. It has a quick onset and short duration of action. It is commonly available as 0.5, 1, or 2 per cent. Use 1 per cent with or without adrenaline 1:200 000 This prolongs its action and reduces bleeding. It is safe to use adrenaline in the hand except for the digits.

The safe total dose of lignocaine is 4 mg/kg, i.e. 28 ml of 1 per cent lignocaine in a 70 kg adult.

Bupivicaine has a slower onset but longer duration of action. Use 0.25 per cent or 0.5 per cent ± adrenaline.

The safe total dose of bupivicaine is 2.5 mg/kg, i.e. 35 ml of 0.5 per cent bupivicaine in a 70 kg adult.

Local infiltration

The injection can be through the wound or parallel to it to produce a surrounding area of numbness. Aspirate before injecting to ensure that the needle tip is not intravascular. With multiple injections try to make each puncture through a numb area.

Nerve blocks

To determine the area that a nerve block is going to anaesthetize, refer to Chapter 3 on anatomy.

Median nerve at wrist (Fig. 6.1(a))

Inject 1 cm proximal to the proximal wrist crease just ulnar to the FCR tendon, between it and PL tendon. Point the needle proximally and angled about 30° to the skin surface. Push the needle in about 1 cm (the nerve is not very deep) and inject—there should be no resistance. Then withdraw the needle to just below the skin, turn it through 90° and pass it radially, subcutaneously for 2cm and inject more solution while withdrawing. This anaesthetizes the palmar branch of the nerve.

This block will anaesthetize the radial half of the palm and the volar surfaces of the thumb, index, long and half of the ring finger.

Use up to 5ml 1% lignocaine.

Ulnar nerve at the wrist (Fig. 6.1(a))

Inject 1 cm proximal to the proximal wrist crease just radial to the tendon of FCU. Point the needle proximally and angled at about 45° to the skin surface. Push the needle in about 1.5 cm and inject after aspirating. (The

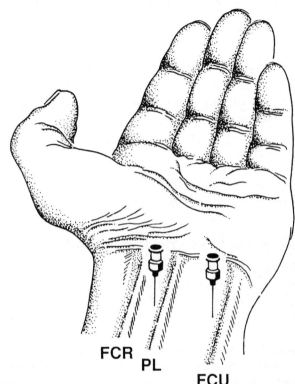

FCR PL FCU

a

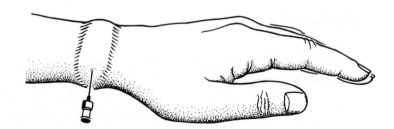

b

Fig. 6.1 • Nerve block at wrist: (a) median or ulnar nerve; (b) radial nerve.

ulnar artery lies next to the nerve on its radial side.) This will block the ulnar half of the palm and the volar aspects of the little finger and half the ring finger. Use up to 5 ml 1 per cent lignocaine.

To block the ulnar half of the dorsal surface of the hand and dorsal surfaces of the little and ring fingers it is necessary to anaesthetize the dorsal branch. Having blocked the ulnar nerve, as above, withdraw the needle to just under the skin, turn it through 90° and pass it towards the ulnar side over the FCU tendon and subcutaneously around the wrist for about 3 cm. Inject 5 ml 1 per cent lignocaine while withdrawing.

Ulnar nerve block at the elbow is not recommended as there is a high incidence of neuritis.

Radial nerve at the wrist (Fig. 6.1(b))

Raise a subcutaneous wheal of local anaesthetic over the snuff box, just ulnar to the APL tendon, and pass the needle over the tendons of the snuff box (the radial artery passes below these tendons), injecting a fan of anaesthetic. This will anaesthetize the radial aspect of the dorsum of the hand, the dorsum of the proximal compartment of the thumb, and the proximal and middle compartments of the index and middle fingers and half the ring finger. Use up to 5 ml of 1 per cent lignocaine.

Digital nerve block

Thumb
To block the volar surface of the thumb, inject subcutaneously beneath the proximal thumb crease along the whole volar aspect. Here the nerves are superficial and can be palpated. Use 2–3 ml 1 per cent plain lignocaine.

To anaesthetize the whole thumb perform a ring block, i.e. a circumferential subcutaneous infiltration at the same level in the thumb. Use up to 5 ml 1 per cent plain lignocaine.

Fingers

For procedures on either side of the finger the digital nerves on both sides are blocked. The preferred site of injection is the web on the dorsal surface which forms a triangle when the fingers are abducted. A 24G needle is inserted into the middle of the triangle and advanced 1.5 cm in a slightly volar direction and towards the side of the affected digit, whilst palpating the web on the volar surface. Three millilitres of 1 per cent lignocaine is injected while slowly withdrawing the needle. The opposite digital nerve must also be blocked by injecting in the adjacent web space (Fig. 6.2). For the radial border of the index and ulnar border of the little finger, the anaesthetic is injected via the dorsal surface of the proxi-

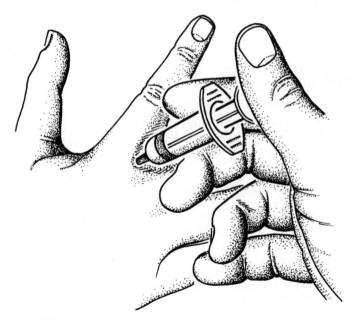

Fig. 6.2• Digital nerve block (ulnar digital nerve to right index finger).

mal compartment, perpendicular to the skin and directed volarly. The needle is advanced until the tip can be felt just deep to the dermis on the volar aspect.

These blocks will only anaesthetize the volar aspect of the fingers and the dorsum from the DIPJ distally. To anaesthetize the dorsal surface of the proximal and middle compartments, inject 1 ml of anaesthetic just below the dermis on each side of the dorsum of the proximal compartment of the finger (one would normally then pass the need volarly to block the volar digital nerve as above).

Bier's block (IV regional anaesthesia)

This is injection of local anaesthetic into the exsanguinated veins of a limb. It is suitable for normotensive adults requiring a closed or open procedure on the forearm or hand that will last for up to an hour. It is a very safe procedure when performed with due care and attention.

Precautions

- Starve and consent as for a GA
- Tipping trolley and full resuscitation equipment
- Monitor patient with ECG and pulse oximeter
- Do not use for patients with vasculitis, sickle cell disease, or crush injury
- Never use Bupivicaine or adrenaline

Note: a second doctor must be available whenever Bier's block is performed.

Technique

- Apply double-cuffed pneumatic tourniquet
- Check patient's blood pressure
- Bilateral venous access (use a small cannula into a small vein on the hand of the affected limb)
- Elevate the limb for 2 minutes to exsanguinate

- Inflate lower cuff (100 mmHg above systolic)
- Inflate upper cuff
- Deflate lower cuff
- Inject 40 ml 0.5 per cent **prilocaine** slowly (over 1–2 minutes)
  NO ADRENALINE
- Inflate lower cuff
- Deflate upper cuff

This produces a sensory block in 10 minutes and a motor block in 20 minutes

DO NOT DEFLATE THE LOWER CUFF AT THE END OF THE PROCEDURE UNTIL IT HAS BEEN INFLATED FOR AT LEAST 25 MINUTES.

Indications of systemic absorption are:
- tingling of lips, tinnitus, bradycardia, hypotension, drowsiness, confusion leading to loss of consciousness, fits.

IF YOU ARE NOT COMPETENT TO MANAGE THESE COMPLICATIONS RAPIDLY AND EFFECTIVELY, THEN IT MAY BE PREFERABLE TO ASK AN ANAESTHETIC COLLEAGUE TO PERFORM A BLOCK.

Other blocks, such as axillary blocks and supraclavicular brachial plexus blocks, are available, but their use should be restricted to experienced anaesthetists and hand surgeons.

Part 2

Soft tissue injuries

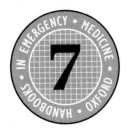

CHAPTER 7

Nail bed injuries

Key points in nail bed injuries

- Significant nail deformity may require later corrective surgery. This may be avoided by the correct primary treatment! A surgical approach is preferred.
- This is a common injury in children—they may need a GA to treat it properly.
- X-rays may not be needed for minor injuries.
- Give antibiotics after trephining if a fracture has not been excluded.

History

Very common presentation to A&E department. Usually a crush injury, trapped in door or between two heavy objects.

Examination

Fingertip is swollen and the nail bed is discoloured with dark blood. The nail plate may be fractured or dislocated, i.e. the proximal part of the nail lies superficial to the eponychial fold. An injury to the underlying nail bed is very common but may not be obvious.

Investigations

X-ray: a fracture of the underlying distal phalanx is common. If there is a fracture of the shaft of the distal phalanx with volar angulation, a laceration of the nail bed is almost inevitable.

Treatment

Digital nerve block and tourniquet (Fig. 6.2). Avulse the nail plate and keep it. Thoroughly clean the wound. Carefully repair the underlying nail bed laceration with 6/0 **absorbable** suture. Suturing the nail bed can be difficult as this tissue tears easily. Take advice from A&E senior or hand surgeon. It is essential to replace the nail under the eponychium to prevent scarring at this site. If the nail is not available or is too damaged, make a false nail from the 'silver' part of the suture packet. The nail or nail substitute may be held in place by the dressings or by a single Steristrip.

Simple dressing with paratulle and gauze.

Antibiotics as it is a compound fracture (flucloxacillin or erythromycin).

A simple subungual haematoma is painful and may become infected. It should be treated by trephining the nail, traditionally with the heated point of a paper clip or a proprietary trephining device. This treatment should be instituted early, but may still be rewarding up to several days after injury.

Referral/follow-up

- Follow up nail bed injuries in A&E review or hand clinic.
- Re-dress at 48–72 hours.

- Advise the patient that the nail will fall off after a few weeks and may be replaced by a new nail, but this takes 3 months to grow out fully. There may be ridging of the nail.
- Displaced fractures of the distal phalanx should be referred for open reduction with repair of the nail bed laceration. A 'step' in the nail bed after healing will prevent nail adherence.
- Have a low threshold for referring children with nail bed injuries for operative repair.

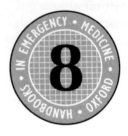

CHAPTER 8

Rupture of the ulnar collateral ligament of the MP joint of the thumb (gamekeeper's thumb)

Key points in UCL rupture

- You may not be able to elicit laxity in fresh injuries because of pain. Refer for senior opinion for tenderness over UCL following a relevant injury.
- Surgery is best performed early if necessary.
- With a complete rupture of the ligament the two ends may come to lie in different anatomical planes and then the ligament will never heal with conservative treatment. This will give a permanently painful and unstable thumb.
- Specifically test for UCL rupture in any thumb injury regardless of the reported mechanism and record your findings.
- An associated avulsion #, if undisplaced, will heal in a Bennett's plaster. Large fragments need ORIF.

History

Fairly common complication of forced abduction of the thumb. Thumb is 'bent back' with a fall. Commonly a skiing injury with the thumb caught in the handle of the ski pole or in the gaps in the surface of a dry ski slope.

Examination

There is swelling of the base of the thumb over the MCP joint and tenderness is present on the ulnar aspect of the joint. Stress the joint into valgus by pulling the thumb with your index and middle fingers with your thumb over the radial aspect of the joint acting as a fulcrum (Fig. 8.1). Is there excess laxity compared with the nor-

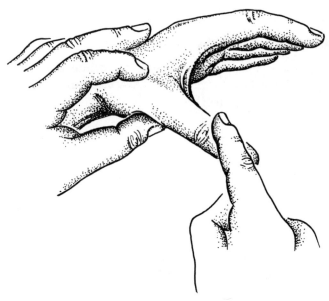

Fig. 8.1 • Testing UCL.

mal side? With a **sprain** there is an increased laxity of the joint for a few degrees but then there is a definite 'stop' to movement. With a **rupture** there is much more laxity, no 'stop', and it feels as though the thumb is going to fall off the metacarpal.

Investigations

X-ray to exclude an associated fracture. If there is doubt about the diagnosis, local anaesthetic can be injected into the site of tenderness and stress X-rays taken.

Treatment

A sprain is treated with an Elastoplast thumb spica. Refer all cases of suspected rupture UCL for assessment by a hand surgeon.

Referral/Follow up

Review sprain after 1 week. Continue Elastoplast spica until tenderness resolves. (Are you sure that it is not a complete rupture?)

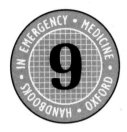

CHAPTER 9

Glass injuries

Key points in glass injuries

- There is often more damage beneath a glass laceration than is clinically suspected.
- All glass is radio-opaque in soft tissue views.
- All deep glass lacerations should be carefully explored.
- Late presenting deeply situated small glass fragments may be treated expectantly in the asymptomatic patient.
- 'Nothing on earth cuts like glass'. Where the patient has fallen onto glass, or glass has fallen onto him, it should be assumed that every structure between skin and bone has been injured.

History

Normally a straightforward history of injury from glass. Ask about loss of movements, loss of sensation, profuse bleeding.

Examination

Glass injuries often produce multiple lacerations. The wounds are typically shelving, at an angle to the skin surface rather than perpendicular. Examine fully for circulation, movement, and sensation. Deep structures may be injured in more than one wound.

Investigations

Always X-ray to exclude a glass FB and injury to bone or joint. Rarely, a thin sliver of glass viewed side-on may be missed radiologically.

Treatment

The treatment of simple lacerations and major injuries are discussed in Chapters 10 and 11 respectively.
Treat bleeding as follows.

- Elevation and direct pressure of gauze and a bandage.
- If severe, use a tourniquet (e.g. a sphygmomanometer cuff inflated above systolic pressure) above the injury. Note the time that the tourniquet is applied. This will also give you an opportunity to inspect the wound briefly whilst it is not bleeding. Release the tourniquet after a pressure bandage is applied.
- Do not use artery clips to clamp the bleeders—you will cause damage to other structures.

Suturing of a shelved wound will give a poor scar; therefore the edges should be minimally excised to give it vertical edges like an incised wound. Refer to a hand surgeon if necessary.

Referral/follow-up

Many glass injuries merit referral. However, if a glass injury appears to be a simple laceration with no underlying damage, it is acceptable to close the wound and reassess the patient after 2–3 days. A nerve or tendon that is found to be divided at this time can be repaired by delayed primary suture.

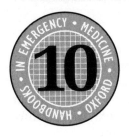

CHAPTER 10

Simple lacerations

Key points in simple lacerations

It is best to leave sutures in the hand longer than elsewhere in the body—thus it allows the patient to mobilize without concern about the wound opening.

History

Usually a straightforward history of a wound from glass or metal. In cases of assault or criminal activity the history may be false. A wound may be self-inflicted.

Examination

Record the length and nature (e.g. ragged) of the wound. Then examine the function of the structures beneath that wound (e.g. nerve, tendon). (See Assessment, Chapter 4.)

Investigations

X-ray for a FB if there is a possibility of a retained piece of glass. Always suspect a FB in glass wounds.

Treatment

Simple non-contaminated lacerations on the hand can be cleaned and sutured under LA using a 4/0 or 5/0 monofilament suture.

Dirty wounds should be cleaned well (usually under LA) and left to heal by 2° intention, or delayed 1° suture at about 3 days if the wound remains clean.

Thorough cleaning is achieved by irrigation with large volumes of saline followed by removal of any residual particulate matter using magnification. Finally, crushed or contaminated wound margins are carefully excised with a 15 scalpel.

If a vital structure (bone, joint, tendon, blood vessel) is exposed in a dirty wound, refer to the hand surgeon for consideration of 1° closure.

Referral/follow-up

Refer all lacerations that are complicated by division of an underlying structure, or are seriously contaminated, to a hand surgeon. For simple lacerations sutures may be removed at 10–14 days.

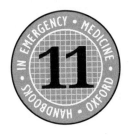

CHAPTER 11

Major lacerations and crush injuries

Key points in major lacerations

- Most bleeding stops with elevation and pressure.
- Beware physiological degloving.
- Do not leave cling film on for more than 1–2 hours as the skin becomes macerated.

History

These injuries can look dreadful, but primary management is straight forward. Ascertain exact nature of injury—what sort of blade, how long limb trapped, any heat involved etc.

Examination

Complete initial assessment and resuscitation of the patient (see p. 147–8). Exclude other more serious injuries and treat these first.

In a severely injured patient, examination of the upper limb is often limited.

Note the general appearance of the limb. Then test the limb for sensation and circulation distally and if possible test movements as well. Further examination is often difficult and of little value acutely.

Physiological degloving

The skin has been pulled off its deep blood supply but there is no wound in the skin. Occurs typically with a tyre rolling over a limb. The skin looks alive but it is not. If you pick the skin up in your fingers it feels unattached to the deep surface. Have a high index of suspicion. Urgent surgery is required.

Investigations

X-ray the injured part.

Treatment

1. IV access—useful for giving IV opioids for analgesia. Small aliquots of morphine (do not give IM opioid to a patient with a major injury). Take blood samples for Hb and cross match.
2. Dress the injury with saline soaked gauze or cling film.
3. Treat bleeding by elevation and direct pressure of gauze and a bandage. If severe, use a tourniquet above the injury. Note the time that the tourniquet is applied and release tourniquet when pressure dressing has been applied. Do not use artery clips to clamp the bleeders—you will cause damage to other structures.

Referral/follow-up

Refer to the hand surgeon.

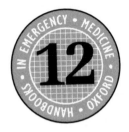

CHAPTER 12

Ring avulsion injury

Key points in Ring avulsion injury

- Ring may be buried under skin flap and not visible. Will show up on X-ray.
- Beware of not assessing the blood supply properly and sending the patient home. The next day the finger may be dead.

History

A spectrum of injuries from simple contusion to complete skin avulsion. Commonly catching a ring on the finger on a hook or similar followed by a traction force. Also excessive tension in a rope wrapped around the finger or thumb.

Examination

- Are the neurovascular structures damaged?
- Test sensation—pen test for sweat (light touch, pinprick).
- Test vascularity: a pink finger has a normal circulation or mild venous congestion—a white finger has no arterial input and low tissue turgor—a blue finger has venous congestion.
- Test tendon function.

Investigations

X-ray to exclude a fracture. This worsens the prognosis considerably.

Treatment

- Remove ring.
- If no skin loss, normal circulation, normal sensation, full ROM, and no fracture—light dressing and mobilize.
- If any complication refer to the hand surgeon.

Referral/follow-up

For a minimal injury review at 48 hours and dress as required. If in any doubt refer to the hand surgeon.

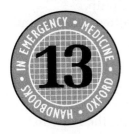

CHAPTER 13

High-pressure injection injuries

Key points in high-pressure injection injuries

- Wound may be very small or not visible
- Suggestive history mandates urgent referral
- Avoid digital nerve blocks and tight dressings

History

Uncommon but important industrial injury frequently affecting the index fingertip of the non-dominant hand. High pressure injection of foreign material (e.g. wax, grease, paint, solvent, oil). The patient has frequently been cleaning the nozzle of a high-pressure gun when material is inadvertently injected.

- May penetrate to deeper structures including the flexor tendon sheath.
- Pressure may cause material to extend proximally as far as the palm.
- Chemical inflammation and secondary infection may lead to tissue necrosis of the whole finger.

Examination

- There may be few early physical signs.

- Usually a tiny entrance wound on the pulp.
- Later on the finger may become swollen, tender, and stiff.

Investigations

X-ray—if the material is visible on X-ray, then the distribution of the material can be seen.

Treatment

- Urgent referral to the hand surgeon for immediate exploration and removal of foreign material.
- Elevate for transfer.

Referral/follow-up

Treatment and follow-up by the hand surgeons.

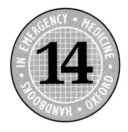

CHAPTER 14

Thermal burns

Key points in thermal burns

- In children always consider non-accidental injury. Small burn + NAI—refer to the paediatricians.
- Do not use Flamazine if the depth of the burn needs to be assessed at 48 hours to consider early surgery. If in doubt, use a paratulle dressing or a plastic bag.
- If the paratulle dressing is adherent to the burn at follow-up, but the wound appears clean and non-infected, leave the paratulle to separate with healing. Repeated tearing off or soaking off the dressing slows healing.

History

May be a scald (bath, radiator steam), contact (iron), or flame. Important to exclude other more serious injuries and smoke inhalation. A detailed history about the mechanism of the burn, length of exposure, and first aid given will help to determine the depth and severity of the burn.

Examination

Observe size and distribution of the burn. Entire palm with closed fingers equals 1% BSA (body surface area). Estimate the depth of the burn.

Estimation of burns depth

Burn depth is difficult to assess at the time of injury even for an experienced clinician.

- Superficial (first-degree)—reddening of the skin—the epidermis is intact and does not peel off if rubbed vigorously. Areas of erythema are not included in estimation of burn size.
- Partial thickness or dermal (second-degree)—intact or broken blisters with a bright red raw surface. Will heal within 2 weeks.
- Deep dermal (second-degree)—may initially look like a superficial burn, but becomes drier with matt red blotches on a paler background, 'salt and pepper' appearance. Will not heal within 2 weeks and leaves a poor scar.

Superficial and dermal burns are painful.

- Full thickness (third-degree)—dry leathery and anaesthetic. May see coagulated vessels in the wound.
- Fourth-degree burns involve deeper structures, e.g. tendon, bone.

Treatment

- Do not forget tetanus prophylaxis.
- Tiny discrete areas may be treated with dressings, e.g. silver sulphadiazine (Flamazine). Superficial burns and scalds may be treated by mobilization within a polythene bag.
- Any significant area of hand burn needs discussion with and probably referral to the hand surgeon.
- If the hand injury is part of a more significant burn elsewhere, then refer to the regional burns unit.

Referral/follow-up

Will need dressings every 2 to 3 days until healed.
Watch out for any stiffness developing, and if necessary
refer to physiotherapy.

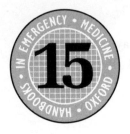

CHAPTER 15

Chemical burns including hydrofluoric acid

Key points in chemical burns

- Seek specific antidote from place of work, if available.
- Alkalis can seem innocuous initially, but they keep burning and may produce a full-thickness burn. They need prolonged washing with water.
- Some chemicals may produce an eczematous reaction that is difficult to distinguish from a burn.
- Chemical powders should be brushed off the skin.
- Irrigation may produce an exothermic reaction.

History

Alkalis are generally worse than acids except for HF. Acids form insoluble protein complexes which are inert. Alkalis form soluble complexes which dissociate, and the anion continues to cause tissue damage. HF also causes deep damage until the fluoride ion is neutralized by Ca^{2+}. The following should be noted:

- Exact nature of chemical.
- Length of exposure.
- If the burn has been washed.
- If a specific antidote has been applied.

Examination

Assess size and distribution of burn.
- Hydrofluoric acid (used for cleaning stone) often attacks the nail beds.

Investigations

With a significant HF burn it is necessary to check plasma Ca^{2+}.

Treatment

- Most chemicals are treated by prolonged dilution with large volumes of water.
- HF burns need initial immediate treatment with the specific cream (calcium gluconate). However, HF produces progressive tissue necrosis and may require neutralization by subcutaneous injection of 10 per cent calcium gluconate.
- **Large HF burns can be fatal.**

Referral/follow-up

Small burns can be managed with simple dressings
- Refer all HF burns to the hand surgeon.
- Refer any burn of significant size.

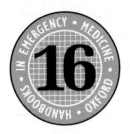

CHAPTER 16

Electrical burns

Key points in electrical burns

- Electrical burns are always deep.
- Clothing may ignite, causing a thermal burn.
- Fasciotomy of severely burned muscle may release myoglobin into the circulation and produce renal failure. IVFR to ensure supranormal urine output.
- Late cardiac complications are a feature of high-voltage injury and do not usually occur following domestic electrocution.

History

- Find out whether the electrical injury was from a domestic supply (240 V 50 MHz) or a high-voltage industrial supply (may be thousands of volts).
- Did clothing ignite?

Examination

- There is usually an entry and exit site burn.
- High-voltage burns (>1000 V) produce massive coagulation of tissue and circulatory problems within the limb.
- Assess distal circulation.
- Estimate size of burn, (palm of patient's hand is approximately 1 per cent of body surface area).

Investigations

- Twelve-lead ECG and monitor.
- Routine haematology and biochemistry including CK and LDH.

Treatment

- Tiny burns, a few millimetres in diameter, may be treated conservatively with silver sulphadiazine (Flamazine).
- Larger discrete burns of the hand/upper limb need referral to the hand surgeon.
- Large burns need referral to a burns unit.
- Patient may require an escharatomy or fasciotomy if the circulation is embarrassed.

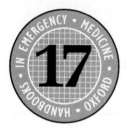

CHAPTER 17

Frostbite

Key points in frostbite

- Prevent stiffness by allowing mobility within the dressings from day 1.
- Very early debridement is not warranted as a surprising amount of healing can take place at the fingertips.

History

- Lesions of the fingertips similar to burn wounds, with a similar classification by depth (see p. 66).
- Follows exposure to low temperatures.
- Not necessarily an ambient temperature of 0°C.

Examination

- Fingers more commonly affected than toes.
- Discrete areas of dead skin on tips.
- Check that there is no cellulitis.

Investigations

- X-ray to see if there is any bone involvement.

Treatment

- Conservative—mobilize in a Flamazine bag, or in small individual dressings.
- Antibiotics for infection or bone involvement.
- Large areas of frostbite may need earlier surgery.

Referral/follow-up

- Small areas will heal with conservative treatment.
- Larger areas may need formal amputation at some stage.
- Significant infection may need admission for IV antibiotics.

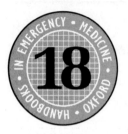

CHAPTER 18

Skin loss

Key points in skin loss

- Small areas of skin loss on the fingertip are treated by the application of a semipermeable film dressing (e.g. Opsite).

(See also fingertip injuries, burns.)

History

- Is there really skin loss, or is it just elastic retraction of the skin edges?
- What structures are beneath the wound?
- Is there any underlying injury?

There is usually an obvious history of cutting, crushing, or avulsion of tissue.

Examination

- Examine for damage to deeper structures—nerve, artery, tendon, bone
- Are there vital structures exposed—tendon, joint, bone?

Investigations

Consider X-ray:

- For opaque FB, if indicated.
- For underlying fracture, if indicated.

Treatment

Small wounds—lavage (with at least 500 ml warm saline) for dirty wounds and close without tension.

Small areas of skin loss (up to 1 cm^2) with no exposed vital structures may be treated conservatively with dressings. The dressing renders the wound pain free and only needs to be changed weekly.

Refer for consideration of graft/flap cover if:

- Extensive tissue loss.
- Any crushing element to the injury.
- The tissue loss crosses a joint crease.
- There is underlying damage.
- There are structures exposed.

Referral/follow-up

Small areas of loss may need weekly dressings for 3–6 weeks to complete healing.

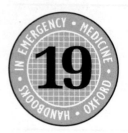

CHAPTER 19

Fingertip injuries

Key points in fingertip injuries

- This is the term used for injuries to the pulp. Nail bed injuries are different (see p. 49).
- Shortening the digit of a small child is bad practice.
- Full-thickness tissue loss of the fingertip may appear to be a trivial injury, but poor management may leave a patient with a prolonged or permanent disability.

History

- Usually a slicing injury.
- May just expose pulp or bone/flexor tendon.
- Initial treatment is very important as this is the best time to obtain a good result from what appears to be a minor injury, but one that can lead to significant morbidity.
- History of cut from glass or knife, or avulsion of tip in door/chain, or crush from a heavy object, e.g. paving stone.

Examination

Determine size of defect and whether bone is exposed.

- Check for a nail bed injury.
- Determine obliquity of injury—the hand surgeon may

enquire whether the injury is transverse, volar oblique, or dorsal oblique (Fig. 19.1).

Investigations

X-ray to look for fracture, crush fracture, or loss of tip of distal phalanx.

Treatment

- Continued minor bleeding can be a problem with slicing injuries of the pulp. It can be treated by application of an alginate dressing which is left undisturbed until the next review.

- Some children (less than 8 years old) may be treated **conservatively** even if a small amount of bone is sticking out. Take senior advice. Simple dressing only (e.g. Opsite).
- Treat defects less than 1 cm^2 with pulp exposure only with simple dressings.
- Refer larger soft tissue defects, or bone exposure, for flap cover/terminalization.

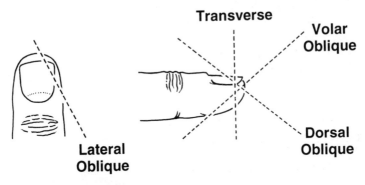

Fig. 19.1 • Fingertip injuries.

- Dressings may be adherent (not to be changed frequently) or non-adherent (changed regularly).
- Undisplaced fractures are usually treated conservatively.
- Antibiotics for compound fractures.
- There is no place for a skin graft—lesions that will not heal spontaneously require a flap.

Referral/follow-up

- Follow-up in review clinic or hand surgery outpatients.
- Children—tell parents that it will take several weeks to heal but this will give the best-looking finger.
- If in doubt, refer to the hand surgeon.

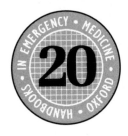

CHAPTER 20

Amputations (replants)—total and subtotal

Key points in amputations

- **TREAT LIFE-THREATENING INJURIES FIRST.**
- Avoid delay ('toxins' are released from anoxic muscle).
- Avoid damage to the amputation stump and the part.
- Refer all cases and let the transplant team discuss with the patient the feasibility/wisdom of replanting.
- **NEVER IMMERSE THE PART IN SALINE.**
- **NEVER PUT THE PART IN DIRECT CONTACT WITH ICE.**

(See also fingertip injuries, degloving injuries.)

History

- May be a guillotine/machete injury producing a clean amputation.
- May be crushed or pressed in a machine producing a large zone of injury. Ask whether the machine is heated (burn plus crush).
- May be an avulsion injury, pulling out the vessels, nerves, or tendons.

Examination

- Examine level and extent of amputation, degree of crush.
- For a partial amputation assess whether there is a distal circulation, sensibility, movement.

Investigations

- X-ray the stump **and the amputated part** (this provides useful information to the replant surgeon).
- Check FBC: cross match two units of PRBC if proximal to fingers, four units if proximal to wrist.

Treatment

- Bleeding is not usually a problem by the time that the patient arrives at the A&E. If it is, apply a BP cuff to the arm and inflate 50 mm above systolic whilst a dressing is applied. Keeping the limb elevated after letting down the cuff will normally prevent further bleeding.
- Set up IV with a 16G cannula (on another limb), take blood samples, and give analgesia, antibiotics, and tetanus toxoid if necessary.
- Simple dressing for the stump e.g. paratulle, cling film.
- Place amputated part in saline-moistened swab in a polythene bag. Lay this on top of ice in a container.
- **NEVER IMMERSE THE PART IN SALINE.**
- **NEVER PUT THE PART IN DIRECT CONTACT WITH ICE.**

Referral/follow-up

Transfer to the microsurgical centre as soon as the patient is fit to travel (see Chapter 6).

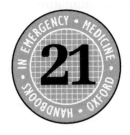

CHAPTER 21

Foreign body in fingertip

Key points in foreign body in fingertip

- If the patient feels that there is a FB present, then there usually is.
- Beware the incomplete removal of foreign body by the patient or doctor.
- Cut the barb off a fishing hook or remove it antegradely (forward).

History

- Common injury—materials include wood splinters, thorns, glass, and metal, including fishing hooks.
- Patient may present late and may have attempted removal himself.
- Almost all isolated FBs require exploration and removal.
- The key to successful removal is a bloodless field.
- Enquire exact nature of injury and material.
- Present symptoms.
- Any treatment to date.

Examination

- Non-irritant foreign material may present with tenderness only or visible signs of penetration of the skin.

- Vegetable matter causes signs of local inflammation or infection with redness, swelling, and possibly purulent discharge.
- Examine specifically for a deep-space infection or purulent tenosynovitis (see Chapter 42).

Investigations

X-ray with soft tissue penetration in two planes may reveal the nature and site of the FB.

In some centres, interested radiologists will perform an ultrasound scan for a wooden or plastic FB. This technique is operator dependent with variable sensitivity and specificity.

Treatment

1. Digital nerve block (see p. 43).
2. Exsanguinate the finger (see p. 33).
3. Follow the track of the FB by sharp dissecting scissors.
4. Remove FB.
5. Through irrigation with warm saline.
6. Dressing and elevation.
7. Antibiotics (e.g. flucloxacillin).
8. Review at 48 hours.

Part 3

Tendon and nerve injuries

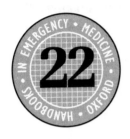

CHAPTER 22

Flexor tendons

FPL to thumb
FDS and FDP to each finger
FCU, FCR, and PL at the wrist
(see Anatomy, Chapter 3)

Key points in flexor tendon injuries

- In some individuals the little finger has no functioning FDS tendon
- The FDP tendon of the index finger is independent of the other FDP tendons. When testing FDS to the index, confirm that the DIPJ is floppy (see Assessment, Chapter 4).
- Beware the partially-cut flexor tendon which snaps a few days later. Take senior advice on suspicion.

History

- Usually a laceration, although may occasionally be a closed rupture (particularly FDP).
- May be secondary to a fracture—then difficult to diagnose as pain may inhibit movement.
- Most commonly a glass or knife wound.

Examination

Examine tendons individually (see Assessment, Chapter 4). If both flexors to a finger are cut, the finger will remain straight and only flex at the MPJs on making a fist (action of lumbrical muscles). If just the FDP is cut the finger will flex at the PIPJ but not at the DIPJ. Partial tendon cut may be suspected if there is pain on resisted flexion.

Look for associated nerve injury (see p. 28).

Assess circulation to digit (see p. 30).

Investigations

X-ray to exclude FB where indicated.

In a closed rupture X-ray may reveal avulsion of FDP insertion at the base of the distal phalanx. On the lateral or oblique film you will see a small fragment of bone volar to the middle phalanx sitting free within the flexor sheath.

Treatment

All flexor tendons should be referred for primary repair by the hand surgeon as post-operative rehabilitation is very important. The surgeon repairing a flexor tendon needs to supervise the patient himself for 8 weeks.

If there is going to be a delay before repair by the hand service, then the wound should be lavaged, sutured, and splinted.

Referral/follow-up

- These injuries are managed by the Hand Surgery service.
- Protective splint for up to 8 weeks.
- Physiotherapy for 12 weeks or more.

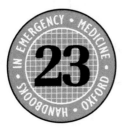

CHAPTER 23

Extensor tendons 1 —mallet finger

Key points in mallet finger

- Make sure that the PIPJ is free to move in the splint.
- Skin care is difficult to maintain.
- Make sure that the patient does not remove the splint and bend the finger. The splint can be removed to wash and dry the finger, but the finger must be supported on a flat surface while the splint is off.
- Some residual extension lag is common even after the best treatment and should be accepted. A significant deformity may be improved by immobilization for a further 6 weeks.

History

- Disruption of the extensor tendon to the terminal phalanx.
- Presents with inability to extend the DIPJ.
- Occurs with trauma, typically to the end of the finger.
- Can also be very minor or forgotten trauma.
- May complicate laceration over DIPJ.

Examination

DIPJ held flexed: full **passive** extension.

Investigations

X-ray to look for fracture at base of distal phalanx.

Treatment

- Closed, spontaneous (no fracture): mallet splint for 6 weeks—refer to hand surgeon.
- Fracture: may need operative treatment for large fragment—Refer to hand surgeon.

Referral/follow-up

- First review within 1 week to check that the splint fits, the skin is not macerated, and PIPJ is moving. Then review fortnightly.
- Refer to physiotherapy for skin care advice.
- After splint is removed tell patient to mobilize slowly but not force it. Movements will improve with time.

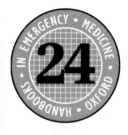

Extensor tendons 2 —division of extensor tendon over proximal phalanx (boutonnière deformity)

Key points in boutonnière deformity

- Commonly missed injury.
- Tell patient to return if finger starts to flex at the PIPJ and he cannot straighten it fully. Then refer to hand clinic.

History

May be an open or a closed injury causing a division of the central slip of the extensor tendon:

- Closed injury, following a sudden forced flexion—rugby injury
- Open injury—knife/glass

Examination

- Often painful.
- May initially have full extension at PIPJ (due to lateral slips functioning) and only develop the boutonnière deformity after a few days or weeks.
- Occasionally may present as an acute boutonnière.
- Test PIPJ for stability of collateral ligaments as this is a more serious injury.

Investigations

X-ray closed injuries to look for a pull-off # where the central slip of the extensor tendon inserts into the base of middle phalanx. Sometimes, because of soft tissue swelling, the X-ray provides the first evidence of a developing boutonnière deformity.

Treatment

- Open injury—needs operative repair. Refer to hand surgeon.
- Closed injury—if recognized as a central slip injury needs specialized splintage of the PIPJ, allowing the MPJ and DIPJ to mobilise. Refer to hand surgeon.

Referral/follow-up

- Difficult injury.
- Best if followed up by hand surgeon.
- Bring a patient with a swollen PIPJ that extends fully, back to A&E after 2–3 days to review.

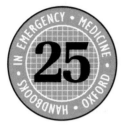

CHAPTER 25

Extensor tendons 3 —division of extensors over MPJs

Key points

- Danger of septic arthritis if a tooth wound is missed. Patients often deny this part of the history. Ask them specifically and tell them that its important.
- Forced abduction of a finger sometimes produces a tear of the sagittal band with volar dislocation of the extensor tendon. It presents with some loss of extension at the MPJ. This injury should be referred for repair.

History

- May be secondary to a human bite or punch to teeth
- Usually an open injury

Examination

Diagnosis may be difficult as there may still be good extension of the MPJ. The sagittal bands at the side of the tendons may be sufficient to effect some extension. (Note that PIPJ and DIPJ will still extend due to action of intrinsic muscles.)

Investigations

X-ray of MPJs if a human bite. Brewerton views show MC heads best. May see piece of tooth or small flake off MC head.

Treatment

- Operative repair of the tendon. Refer to hand surgeon.
- Need to wash out MPJ if opened.
- Splint (volar POP slab) with MPJ at 0° allowing movement of PIPJ and DIPJ.

Referral/follow-up

- Follow-up weekly.
- Remove splint at 3 weeks and mobilize.

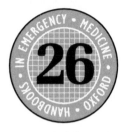

CHAPTER 26

Extensor tendons 4 —division of extensors over dorsum of hand and wrist

Key points

- Extensor tendons are flat and therefore it is difficult to use a Kessler-type core stitch. Two 3/0 or 4/0 vicryl horizontal mattress sutures are adequate.
- Non-absorbable sutures may show through the thin skin over the repair.

History

- Usually an open injury.
- Rheumatoid patient may present with spontaneous rupture.
- Rupture of EPL may occur after a Colles' fracture.

Examination

- Look at the cascade of the fingers at rest (Fig. 4.1).
- Extensor division will cause drooping of the affected finger.

- Test extension at MPJs (PIPJs and DIPJs will extend due to the action of the intrinsic muscles).

Investigations

Soft tissue X-ray to exclude glass FB if indicated.

Treatment

- Primary repair of extensor tendons. Refer to hand surgeon.
- Static splintage for 3 weeks with wrist dorsiflexed.
- MPJs at 70°–90° and IPJs straight. It is safe to hold the MPJs flexed as the wrist is dorsiflexed.

Referral/follow-up

May need physiotherapy after splintage.

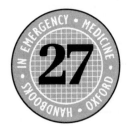

CHAPTER 27

Nerve injuries

Key points in nerve injuries

- If you do not think that the nerve is injured, and there are no other injuries, it is very acceptable to close the wound (suture or tapes) and review the patient at 48 hours. If a nerve division is confirmed at this time, a delayed primary suture can be performed.

History

- Usually a laceration or incised wound.
- A nerve injury may be associated with a fracture.
- Numbness with a closed injury is often due to nerve contusion (neuropraxia).

Examination

With any laceration or wound, think which structures are in this area and test the relevant nerves. Make a specific examination of the median, ulnar, radial and digital nerves (see Assessment, Chapter 4).

Beware of false negatives. A patient with a divided nerve may occasionally still have sensation for some hours.

Treatment

Any nerve injury should be considered for repair using microsurgical technique and magnification. Refer to the hand surgeon.

Referral/follow-up

Refer all nerve injuries to a hand surgeon. Although not all nerve injuries are repaired, this is a decision for a hand surgeon based on a number of factors: which nerve, which finger, which hand; age and occupation of the patient and the time since injury. Nerve repair does not always restore function but will usually prevent the development of a painful neuroma.

Part 4

Injuries to bones and joints

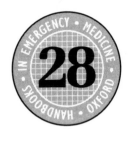

CHAPTER 28

Fall on outstretched hand (FOOSH)

Key points on FOOSH

- May miss an associated injury to the elbow or shoulder.
- Scaphoid fractures may be difficult to diagnose (see p. 101).
- Why did the patient fall?

History

Common injury in elderly women and young men. Pain in the wrist after a fall. Exact mechanism of injury often not recalled.

Examination

- Look for swelling and deformity.
- Palpate the lower forearm, wrist, ASB, and hand carefully to elicit exactly the point of maximum tenderness.
- Test movements of thumb, fingers, and wrist to check integrity of tendons (? closed rupture) and to assess where the pain is on movement.

Investigations

X-rays. AP and lateral of wrist, plus others if indicated by examination (e.g. scaphoid views or hand X-ray).

Treatment

Depends on the diagnosis. The following diagnoses are discussed elsewhere:

- Fracture of MC base (p. 110).
- Scaphoid fracture (p. 101).
- Lunate dislocation and scapho-lunate dissociation (p. 104).
- Colles' and Smith's fractures are dealt with in other textbooks, and there is usually a departmental policy agreed with the orthopaedic department.

In most other cases there is just a soft tissue injury or sprained wrist. Other rare injuries (e.g. fracture of pisiform or hamate) are usually treated conservatively. A crepe bandage may give some psychological support and serves as a reminder to others that this person has a sore wrist.

Referral/follow-up

Sprained wrists are common. Very few go on to give chronic wrist pain. Symptoms should subside in a few days to a fortnight. If symptoms are not improving or continue after 2 weeks, refer to a hand surgeon. An unusual diagnosis may have been missed or the patient may have an injury that will proceed to chronic wrist pain.

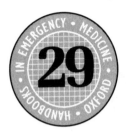

CHAPTER 29

Scaphoid fracture

Key points on scaphoid fractures

- An easy fracture to miss.
- Delayed treatment may cause delayed union or non-union.
- Beware an associated dislocation of the lunate, scapho-lunate dissociation, and other injuries to the carpus.
- A fracture of the distal end of the radius may present with tenderness in the ASB.
- Fractures of the radius and scaphoid may occur following the same injury.

History

- Usually occurs in young males.
- Very rare in children.
- Fall on dorsiflexed wrist or kickback from a starting handle. May follow minimal force in an osteopenic wrist. (See Fig. 29.1.)

Examination

- Fullness in the ASB (not reliable).
- Tenderness in the ASB.
- Tenderness on pressing the scaphoid tubercle. This bony prominence lies volarly, just distal to the lower

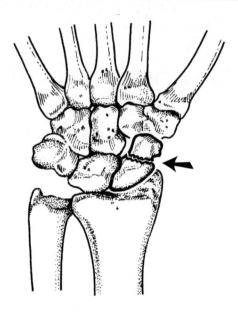

Fig. 29.1 • Fractured waist of scaphoid (arrow).

end of the radius, and is most easily palpated in the radially deviated wrist. This is a good test so it is worth practising palpation of the scaphoid tubercle.
- Pain on axial compression of the thumb.
- Carefully examine the rest of the hand and wrist.

Investigations

Scaphoid view X-rays. Four views are usually taken: AP, lateral, and two obliques.

Treatment

With the typical history and tenderness in the ASB, treat with a 'scaphoid' POP whether or not there appears to be a fracture. Your department may have alternative policy for 'clinical scaphoids'.

Referral/follow-up

- If no fracture on first X-ray, review at 2 weeks. X-ray again with POP off—if still tender but no fracture, replace POP and refer to fracture clinic.
- Refer fractures to the next fracture clinic.
- Displaced fractures should be referred early as internal fixation may be the treatment of choice.
- Clinically positive, repeated X-ray-negative 'query scaphoids' may represent intercarpal ligament disruption. Refer to a hand surgeon.

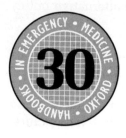

CHAPTER 30

Intercarpal ligament disruption: lunate dislocation and scapho-lunate dissociation

Key points

- Pain and swelling are often severe, X-rays may look relatively normal.
- Median nerve may be involved by direct contusion or later swelling. May need acute decompression of the median nerve.
- Look for concomitant injuries from this high-energy trauma—CMC dislocation, radio/ulnar dislocation, elbow dislocation, radial head fracture.

History

- Occurs with or without a scaphoid fracture.
- There may be a fracture of the radial styloid.
- Extreme hyperextension injury of the wrist such as a fall from a height or a motorcycle injury.

Examination

- Wrist is held in neutral position.
- Swelling may be only moderate.

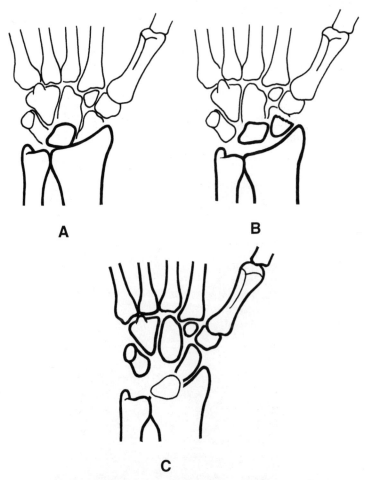

Fig. 30.1 • Perilunate injuries. Appearance of wrist: on AP X-rays: bold outline, bones in normal anatomical plane; light outline, bones displaced relative to normal position. (Modified, with permission from McRae (1994) *Practical fracture treatment*, Churchill-Livingstone.)

- There is diffuse tenderness of the wrist.
- ROM is significantly decreased by pain.
- Examine median nerve function (see p. 29).

Investigations

X-ray wrist—AP, lateral, and scaphoid views. Look at the lunate on the lateral X-ray. Remember that any of the following may be associated with a scaphoid fracture (Fig. 30.1):

- perilunate dislocation (A)
- scapho-lunate dissociation (B)
- volar lunate dislocation (C)

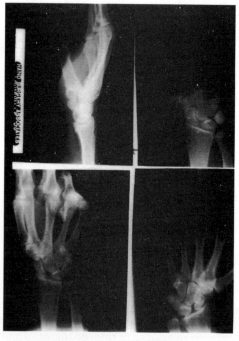

Fig. 30.2 • X-rays of wrist. Clenched fist view (bottom left) shows scapho-lunate dissociation.

On the PA view the lunate looks more triangular than its usual trapezoid shape. X-rays can be very difficult to interpret. Carpal instability may be dynamic and not show on an X-ray. A clenched fist view may show widening of the gap between the scaphoid and the lunate (Fig. 30.2).

Treatment

Volar slab and broad arm sling prior to immediate transfer.

Referral/follow-up

- Lunate dislocation: refer to hand surgeon for closed or open reduction.
- Wrist pain following a severe force and no obvious bony injury should be referred to the hand surgery clinic.

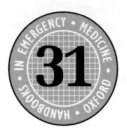

CHAPTER 31

Bennett's fracture

Key points on Bennett's fracture

- Poor reduction may lead to prolonged pain and early arthritic changes.

History

A fracture of the articular surface of the base of the thumb metacarpal. The small fragment remains in place. The rest of the metacarpal is subluxed owing to the pull of the EPB tendon (Fig. 31.1(a)).

The fracture is caused by a longitudinal compression force to the thumb combined with a torsion or angulatory force.

Examination

- Swelling and tenderness may be mild.
- Direct pressure over the fracture, just distal to the ASB, causes pain.

Investigations

X-ray of thumb.

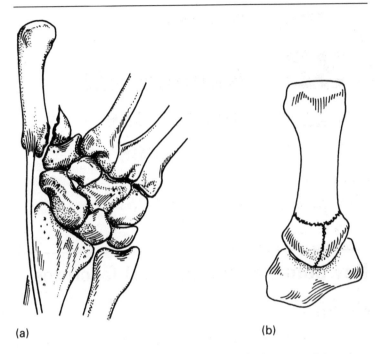

(a)   (b)

Fig. 31.1 • (a) Bennett's fracture; (b) Rolando fracture of thumb MC.

Treatment

- Closed reduction is difficult to maintain in a POP.
- Refer to hand surgeon for closed or open reduction.
- Reduction needs to be maintained for 6 weeks.
- Crepe bandage and sling for transfer to hand surgeon.

A Rolando fracture of the first MC base should be referred to the hand surgeon for pinning or ORIF (Fig. 31.1(b)).

Referral/follow-up

Refer to hand surgeon.

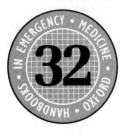

CHAPTER 32

Metacarpal shaft/base fractures

Key points on metacarpal fractures

- Look for dislocation at CMCJ if there is fracture of the base of MC.

History

May occur from a punch or a direct blow to the hand. **Patients are often very economical with the truth when describing the mechanism of injury.**

Examination

Slight swelling. Tenderness at site of fracture. Loss of knuckle on flexion of MPJs with shaft fractures. Check if there is rotation or angulation of the fingers, i.e. observe during slow active flexion, looking for scissoring, and look at the nails end on for rotation, (Fig. 32.1(a)).

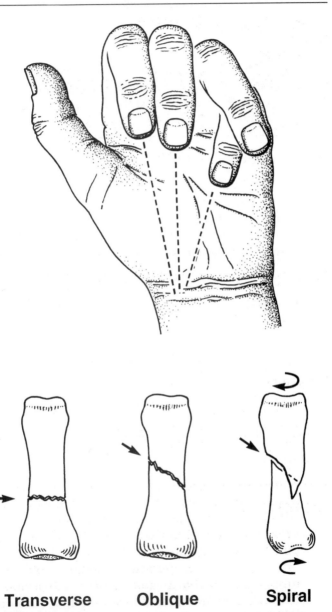

(a)

(b)

Transverse   **Oblique**   **Spiral**

Fig. 32.1 • (a) Scissoring caused by rotation/angulation of a fractured proximal phalanx; (b) metacarpal fractures.

Investigations

X-ray hand. Look for the site of fracture. Do not forget that there may be more than one fracture. Note type of fracture—oblique, transverse, spiral, etc. (Fig. 32.1(b)). Is there any displacement of the fragments?

Treatment

- If the fracture is stable and undisplaced with no rotation, neighbour strap and mobilize.
- If it is an unstable fracture (oblique or spiral) or if there is rotation, angulation, or significant displacement, refer to hand surgeon as it may need internal fixation.

Referral/follow-up

- Review stable fractures at 1 week. If there is no change clinically, continue neighbour strapping for a further 2 weeks.
- If you are unhappy about the hand, repeat X-ray to check the fracture position.

Stability

Some experience is required before any hand fracture is described as stable. Generally, stable fractures are single with minimal displacement and angulation. They do not extend into the joint. In addition, consider whether the pull of related tendons will cause further displacement or angulation, e.g. Bennett's fracture. Stable hand fractures are generally treated by early active mobilization. Unstable fractures should be referred for consideration of ORIF.

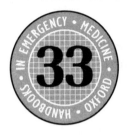

CHAPTER 33

Fractured neck of fifth metacarpal

Key points on fractured neck of fifth MC

- Ask patient specifically if a punch on a tooth occurred.
- At follow-up check extension lag, i.e. loss of full extension of the little finger, and encourage extension exercises.
- This fracture is different from a shaft or head fracture. Much less angulation is acceptable in shaft fractures, which often need ORIF.
- Fractures of the metacarpal head are intra-articular and need assessment by a hand surgeon.

History

Usually from punching someone or something.

Examination

- Usually closed but may be open, particularly from a punch that strikes the teeth.
- Tender at site of fracture, swollen, loss of knuckle when making a fist.
- May have an extension lag (loss of full extension).

Investigations

X-ray of hand. Can estimate angulation on lateral film. Look also at fourth MC neck for a fracture.

Treatment

If angulation is 30° or less, neighbour strap and mobilize. If very tender, apply a volar slab POP for a few days.

If angulation is more than 30°, consider reduction. Wrist block or fracture block may be adequate analgesia for the procedure. Reduce fracture using thumb pressure on volar aspect of MC head. Volar slab POP. Repeat X-ray to check position. If no improvement, refer to hand surgeon.

It is frequently suggested that any degree of angulation is acceptable with a MC neck fracture. This is incorrect. Neglected angulated neck fractures lead to a lump in the palm (MC head) which may be tender when gripping an object.

Referral/follow-up

- Neighbour strapping is maintained for 7 days.
- A volar slab may be removed after a few days and replaced with neighbour strapping for 7 days.
- After closed reduction, a volar slab is worn for 2 weeks before mobilizing in neighbour strapping.

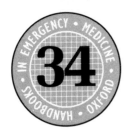

CHAPTER 34

Phalangeal fractures

Key points on phalangeal fractures

- Fractures treated in A&E must be kept under review to ensure that stiffness does not develop—may need to refer to physiotherapy.

History

- Most common of all hand fractures. The majority are stable injuries.
- Aim is to allow early movement to prevent stiffness.
- Usually caused by a direct blow to the bone or to the end of the finger (axial force), or a hyperextension or hyperflexion injury.

Examination

Painful swollen digit with decreased movements. Check for rotation or angulation caused by the fracture (Fig. 34.1(a)). Look at the fingertips end on with the MPJs at 90° and the IPJs at 0°—this will show any rotation. Then ask the patient to flex the fingers—angulation will cause scissoring (Fig. 32.1(a)).

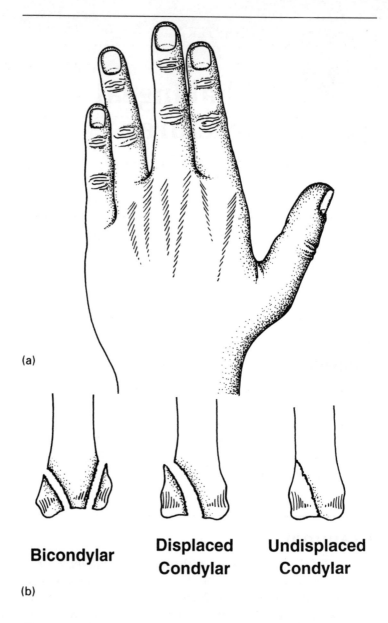

(a)

Bicondylar   **Displaced
Condylar**   **Undisplaced
Condylar**

(b)

Fig. 34.1 • (a) Angulation from fracture of proximal phalanx of
ring finger; (b) condylar fractures of base of phalanx.

Investigations

X-ray to decide type and stability of fracture, and any displacement.

Treatment

Stable undisplaced fractures can be neighbour strapped for 3 weeks and mobilized.

X-rays during this period will not show any callus and are only of value to check that there has not been any displacement of the fracture.

Referral/follow-up

Fractures that need to be referred to the hand surgeon for consideration of internal fixation are:

- angulated shaft fracture
- oblique fracture—this will shorten further and rotate
- any condylar or intra-articular fracture
- severely comminuted fracture
- open fracture.

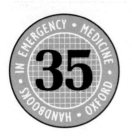

CHAPTER 35

Interphalangeal joint dislocation

Key points on IPJ dislocation

- Warn patient about possibility of flexion contracture after a volar plate injury.

History

- Dorsal dislocation of the PIPJ is most common. May have been reduced by the time the patient attends A&E.
- In describing fractures and dislocations, the direction of the angulation or displacement refers to the movement of the distal fragment.
- Common sport or fighting injury with twisting of the finger. Patient can often feel that the joint is 'out'.

Examination

The finger may look dislocated. The joint is swollen and has markedly reduced movement. A dislocation may not be obvious if it presents late, owing to the swelling.

Investigations

X-ray before manipulation, otherwise you may be

accused of causing the associated fracture. X-ray after manipulation.

Treatment

Reduction under digital nerve block (if there is no fracture)

Technique: extend the joint further, applying slight traction. Then pull very firmly on the finger and pull the middle phalanx over the head of the proximal phalanx into position. The joint is usually quite stable then—test that it has a full range of flexion and repeat X-ray to check position. Test lateral ligament stability. Immobilize PIPJ only (if this is the affected joint) in a Zimmer splint in a few degrees of flexion for 2–3 days to allow the swelling to reduce. Then mobilize in neighbour strapping for 2 weeks.

Referral/follow-up

Review range of movements at 2 weeks—may need referral to physiotherapy.

If there is a fracture or if you cannot reduce the dislocation or if the joint is very unstable after reduction, refer to the hand surgeon. May need open reduction and ligament repair.

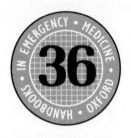

CHAPTER 36

Swollen PIP joint (volar plate injury)

Key points on swollen PIP joint

- Irreversible volar plate contracture (bent finger) can develop late (up to 3 months). Follow up all these injuries at least once. Thereafter, tell the patient to return if the finger starts to bend and will not straighten completely. Then refer to hand surgeon or therapist.
- Warn patient that the swelling of the PIPJ may last for many months or even years.

History

- The volar plate may be injured by hyperextension of the PIPJ.
- Healing may produce fibrosis and shortening of the volar plate leading to a progressive flexion deformity of the PIPJ.
- Usually follows dorsal dislocation or hyperextension of PIP joint of a finger.
- Patient complains of pain, swelling, and stiffness.

Examination

- PIP joint is swollen and therefore usually stable.
- Flexion and extension both present, but a little stiff.

Investigations

X-ray finger to look for pull-off fracture at base of middle phalanx where volar plate inserts (Fig. 36.1) and to check that the joint is fully reduced.

Treatment

Mobilize in neighbour strapping for 3–4 days. A dorsal dislocation is usually easily reduced by hyperextension and longitudinal traction.

Referral/follow-up

Refer to hand surgeon if the pull-off fracture is displaced or if there is marked lateral instability (collateral ligament injury).

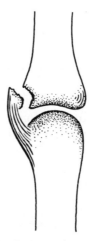

Fig. 36.1 • Volar plate injury with 'pull-off' fracture.

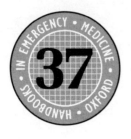

CHAPTER 37

Epiphyseal injuries in children

Key points on Epiphyseal injuries

- The physis is weaker than the ligaments and so is liable to injury.
- Beware missing a type V injury, as it may lead to deformity with growth.
- These are sometimes described as fractures and sometimes as fracture dislocations.
- Fractures heal rapidly in children, and stiffness is unusual.

History

- Hand trapped in door for small children.
- Sports injury in older child.

Examination

May be difficult to detect the injury clinically. A young child may just not be using the hand. May just be some soft tissue swelling.

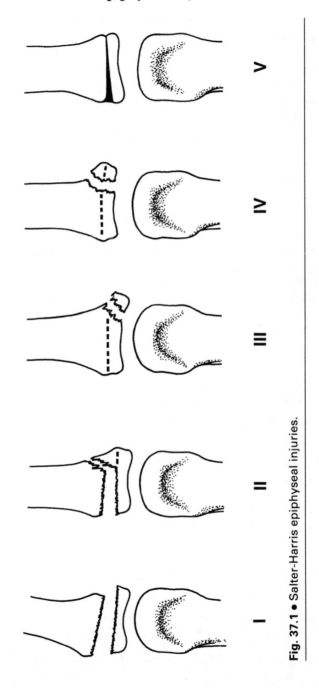

Fig. 37.1 • Salter–Harris epiphyseal injuries.

Investigations

- X-ray of finger: AP, lateral, and an oblique view may be useful to evaluate the injury fully.
- Salter and Harris classification of epiphyseal fractures (see Fig. 37.1).

Treatment

- Place patient's hand and forearm in a volar slab in the safe position until seen by a hand surgeon (same day or next morning).
- Salter and Harris I and II: closed reduction is usually successful, but may need ORIF.
- Older children may be suitable for LA but most will need a GA.
- Type III injury that is significantly displaced and type IV need ORIF.
- Type V injury may need simple immobilization, or manipulation if angulated.

Referral/follow-up

All epiphyseal injuries should be reviewed by a hand surgeon.

Part 5

Infections

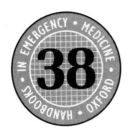

CHAPTER 38

Paronychia

Key points on paronychia

- May spread, if neglected, to infect the pulp space (pulp abscess) or flexor tendon sheath (purulent tenosynovitis).
- Chronic resistant paronychia is often due to fungal infection. Treat by removal of part or all of nail plate, send specimen for culture and prescribe an antifungal cream.
- Consider a malignancy (squamous cell carcinoma, malignant melanoma) in an unusual chronic paronychia.

History

- Common abscess of the nail fold, sometimes spreading under the nail plate.
- Spontaneous development of a painful swelling of the side of the finger nail.

Examination

- Periungal tissues are swollen and red.
- May be evidence of frank pus.

Investigations

- Test urine for sugar
- Pus swab for culture

Treatment

Simple erythema may respond to antibiotics, e.g. coflu-ampicil.

Fluctuant abscess should be drained under digital nerve block, either by developing the space between the nail fold and the nail plate, or by an incision over the area of maximum fluctuance. A large cavity should be packed with ribbon gauze soaked in saline, Betadine cream, or proflavine cream.

Referral/follow-up

Change dressing at 48-hour intervals until healed. This can be done by A&E staff, the practice nurse, or the district nurse.

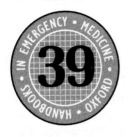

CHAPTER 39

Pulp space infection

Key points on pulp space infection

- Beware of unusual looking or chronic infections. Consider osteomyelitis, foreign body, or squamous cell carcinoma.

History

- Deep infection of the soft tissues of the fingertip usually due to *Staph. aureus* or coliforms.
- Entrapment of pus between the fibrous septa of the pulp causes extreme pain and tenderness of the finger.
- Short history of severe pain and swelling of the tip of the finger.

Examination

Fingertip is swollen, red, and extremely tender.

Investigations

- X-ray to exclude a foreign body and to look for bony involvement.
- After incision send pus for culture and sensitivity.

Treatment

Incision and drainage via a mid-lateral approach (Fig. 3.2, p. 9) or directly through an area that is pointing. Swab for C&S. Thorough irrigation. Pack with ribbon gauze soaked in aqueous Betadine or proflavine. Finger dressing. Five-day course of antibiotics (cofluampicil or erythromycin). Elevate in high sling. Encourage the patient to mobilize the fingers.

Referral/follow-up

Change dressing and review at 48 hours. Change dressing every 2–3 days until healed.

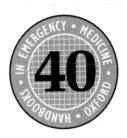

CHAPTER 40

Cellulitis

Key points in cellulitis

- Consider admission for IV antibiotics

History

- Streptococcal infection of the skin and subcutaneous tissues.
- Patient presents with a spreading area of redness and tenderness on the hand or forearm. There may or may not be a history of injury, a puncture wound, or a scratch.
- Possible malaise.

Examination

Local warmth, redness, tenderness, and swelling. Patient may be pyrexial and unwell. Look for ascending lymphangitis (a red streak going up the limb) and for tender adenopathy (supratrochlear at the elbow, and axilla).

Investigations

- Urine for sugar.
- Swab for culture where applicable.

Treatment

- Elevate in sling.
- Oral penicillin or erythromycin for 7 days.
- Admit for IV antibiotics if patient is unwell, if there is lymphangitis or lymphadenopathy, or if there is not a rapid response to oral antibiotics (24 hours).

Referral/follow-up

If not admitted, review at 24 hours by GP or A&E review.

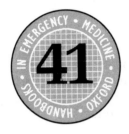

CHAPTER 41

Bite wounds

Key points in bite wounds

- Do not miss the tooth injury to the MPJ of the little finger. It is a common injury and if neglected may lead to complete destruction of the joint.

History

Common presentation, especially dog bites, human bites, and occasionally other animals. The bites are often deep and are inevitably infected.

Often presents late. Patient often does not admit that the injury is a human bite. May be caused by a punch, striking the fifth metacarpal head against teeth!

Examination

Deep ragged wound. May be infected. If the wound is over the fifth metacarpal head, ask very specifically about the mechanism of the injury. If a deep structure has been penetrated, there may be a septic arthritis or tenosynovitis.

Investigations

X-ray for underlying bony injury and retained foreign bodies (tooth fragments). Swab for culture and sensitivity.

Streptococci and mixed anaerobes are the commonest infections. Dogs and cats may harbour *Pasteurella spp.*, and it may cause a serious, spreading infection but is usually sensitive to penicillin.

Human bite wounds from assailants known to be at risk of Hepatitis B infection necessitate an accelerated Hepatitis B vaccination serum for the victim, first draw blood for HBsAg and save serum. Refer to microbiology consultant for advice.

Treatment

Wounds with no underlying deep injury may be treated by debridement and thorough irrigation with warm saline. The wound edges should be trimmed, but the wound should not be sutured unless there is exposure of bone, joint, tendon, or artery. Such cases should be referred. Give antibiotics (co-amoxiclav). Antiseptic dressing if the wound is not closed. Elevate.

Refer all other wounds for exploration, debridement, and irrigation.

If there is tissue loss, refer to hand surgeons.

Referral/follow-up

Simple wounds should be redressed at 48 hours and then every 2–3 days as necessary. Consider a delayed primary closure at 5 days, or leave to heal by secondary intention.

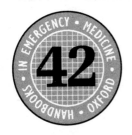

CHAPTER 42

Purulent tenosynovitis

Key points in purulent tenosynovitis

- Pain on passive stretching of the tendon is virtually pathognomonic of purulent tenosynovitis.
- Refer to hand surgeon on suspicion.
- At an early stage IV antibiotics may settle the infection, but it needs constant review as an in-patient.
- Delayed treatment leads to a useless finger.

History

- Infection in a flexor tendon sheath in the finger and palm. Usually *Staph. aureus*; sometimes Gram-negative bacilli, or anaerobes.
- Usually follows a penetrating injury (e.g. a thorn); injury may have been forgotten.
- Rarely, haematogenous spread from focus elsewhere.

Examination

The finger is flexed and held stiff. It is swollen and red. There is tenderness along the line of the tendon. There is no active movement. There may be a little passive movement (differentiates from a septic arthritis). There is exquisite pain on resisted passive extension. The infection may spread into the thenar and mid-palmar spaces of the hand.

Investigations

- Urine for sugar.
- X-ray for a FB.

Treatment

Exploration and drainage usually under GA, antibiotics, immobilization.

Referral/follow-up

Urgent referral to a hand surgeon.

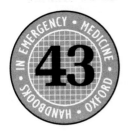

CHAPTER 43

Septic arthritis

Key points in septic arthritis

- An infected joint is usually stiff, and passive movement is not allowed by the patient.
- Refer to the hand surgeon on suspicion.
- Delayed referral may lead to destruction of the articular cartilage.

History

Infection in a joint. Usually MPJ or PIPJ of a finger. Usually following a penetrating injury (e.g. tooth, thorn) which may have been forgotten.

Examination

Red, swollen, warm, tender joint. No active or passive movement present. Patient in a lot of pain if you try and move the joint.

Investigations

- Urine for sugar.
- X-ray for opaque FB and bony changes (osteolysis).
- X-ray may be normal.

Treatment

Refer for drainage and antibiotics.

Referral/follow-up

Urgent referral for surgery.

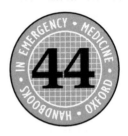

CHAPTER 44

Web space abscess

Key points in web space abscess

- Look for an abscess on both the dorsal and volar surfaces of the web (collar stud). Drain both via a dorsal approach as a volar scar may be tender.
- Don't incise transversely across the web space as this will form a tight scar between fingers.

History

Collection of pus in one of the web spaces in the hand.

May follow a penetrating injury (e.g. thorn). Injury may have been forgotten. May arise from a crack in the skin between the fingers, or track from a subcutaneous infection in the fingers.

Examination

Dorsal and volar swelling, erythema, and pain localized in the web space. The adjacent fingers are abducted.

Investigations

- Urine for sugar.
- X-ray for opaque FB.

Treatment

- Incision dorsally, and pack with ribbon gauze soaked with aqueous Betadine or proflavine.
- Antibiotics.
- Rest and elevation.

Referral/follow-up

Review the patient and change the dressing at 48 hours; then as necessary.

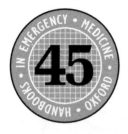

CHAPTER 45

Palmar space infections

Key points in palmar space infections

- Do not just treat with antibiotics and review. Needs immediate assessment by a hand surgeon as delayed or inadequate treatment may lead to a useless hand.
- The tight palmar skin may mean that the abscess presents with swelling under the *dorsal* surface only.

There are potential spaces in the hand where infection can occur. The *mid-palmar space* is deep to the flexor tendons. The *thenar space* lies radial to the third metacarpal. The *hypothenar space* overlies the hypothenar muscles (Fig. 45.1).

History

Arises from a penetrating injury or extension from infection elsewhere in the hand.

Examination

- Mid-palmar space: loss of concavity of palm, dorsal swelling, tender over mid-palmar space, movement of middle and ring fingers is painful and limited.
- Thenar space: swelling over the thenar eminence and first web space, the thumb is abducted.

141

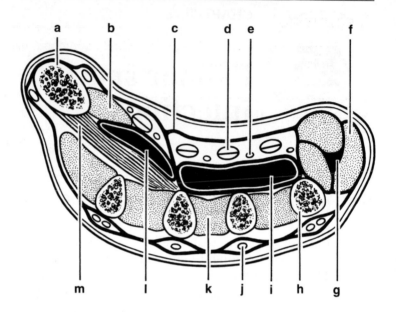

a   thumb MC
b   thenar muscles
c   palmar aponeurosis
d   flexor tendons
e   neurovascular bundle
f   hypothenar muscles
g   hypothenar space

h   fifth MC
i   mid-palmar space
j   extensor tendon
k   interosseous muscles
l   thenar space
m   adductor pollicis

Fig. 45.1 • Spaces of the hand.

- Hypothenar space: rare, swelling and tenderness over the hypothenar eminence.

Investigations

- Urine for sugar.
- X-ray for opaque FB.

Treatment

Exploration and drainage by hand surgeon, usually under GA. Antibiotics.

Referral/follow-up

These conditions are managed by the Hand Surgery service.

Part 6

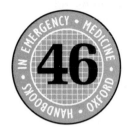

CHAPTER 46

Preparation for patient transfer

Many straightforward hand conditions are adequately dealt with in A&E. More serious problems require assessment by an experienced hand surgeon who may be an orthopaedic or plastic surgeon based in your hospital or in a specialized unit elsewhere.

It is essential to recognize when you are dealing with a problem beyond your experience and to refer appropriately. Some conditions clearly necessitate immediate referral such as amputations of digits or hands. Others may be less obvious, yet are equally important threats to full recovery of function. Examples are high-pressure injection injuries, physiological degloving, and wounds causing vascular compromise. Tendon and nerve lacerations are easily overlooked at first presentation. These types of injuries may legitimately be reviewed at 24–48 hours and referred if necessary at this stage.

Therefore patient transfers are made in a variety of circumstances—sometimes immediate, sometimes later. The transfer may be internal, i.e. within your hospital, or to a distant unit. Whatever the circumstance of the transfer the same basic principles apply.

Resuscitation

In the context of major or multiple injuries, the first priority is to secure the patient's airway and provide high-flow oxygen via a face mask with reservoir. Immediately life-threatening injuries are dealt with first. Two large-bore cannulae should be sited in large veins on unin-jured limbs and blood drawn for routine tests and cross-matching. The remainder of the resuscitation will depend upon the patient's precise injuries and will be guided by the trauma team leader.

Trauma to the extremities, no matter how dramatic in appearance, should be managed after completion of the primary survey and resuscitation phase.

Primary care of the hand injury

Heavy bleeding should be controlled by elevation and direct pressure. This forms part of the resuscitation phase. Exceptionally, if the bleeding is difficult to con-trol, apply a blood pressure cuff to the arm and inflate to 250 mmHg. A brief examination of the wound may now be possible and then a firm dressing can be applied. Place the arm in high elevation and deflate the cuff. Do not explore the wound or attempt to apply haemostats—you will damage vital structures.

Remove any rings.

Dirty lacerations should be irrigated with sterile saline.

Prior to transfer, a simple non-adherent dressing should be applied, e.g. tulle gras covered with saline-soaked gauze. A crepe or cling bandage will hold the dressing in place. Cling film provides an excellent tem-porary dressing for burn wounds. Significant soft tissue injuries or fractures should be immobilized with a volar plaster slab in the position of rest (see p. 36).

To prevent swelling of the hand (which slows healing) the limb should be elevated in a high arm sling.

Opioid analgesia should be given intravenously in doses titrated to response.

Communication

You will need to contact the following prior to transfer.

Hand surgeon

The receiving surgeon will require a clear account of the following:

- patient's name, age, handedness, and occupation
- time of injury, exact mechanism of injury
- precisely which part is injured
- patient's past medical history, medications, and allergies
- time of last meal
- working diagnosis
- investigations to date, and their results
- treatment given to date and response, including IVFR, antibiotics, tetanus prophylaxis
- name of consultant in charge

Receiving A&E

Most patients transferred to another hospital will be taken first to the A&E department. The senior nurse in the A&E department will need to know in advance of the patient's transfer. Details of the patient's condition are required, as well as the name of the receiving surgeon.

Patient's relatives

Anxiety of the patient and his relatives will be allayed by a clear explanation from the referring doctor as to the diagnosis and the reason for transfer to a specialist unit. A&E reception or nursing staff should be able to direct the relatives to the distant hospital. Written instructions are most useful.

Documentation

Ensure that the following accompany the patient:

- clinical records or A&E card or referral letter
- nursing charts

- X-rays (and reports)
- ECG
- Results of laboratory studies
- Blood if cross-matched at the base hospital. Send sufficient blood for the journey only. Multiple units of blood and blood products must not accompany the patient. If not transferred between the *Laboratories* of the referring and receiving hospitals they should not be transfused.

Index